The Menopause Metamorphosis

Transforming with Grace

by
Evelyn Marsh

Table of Contents

Introduction:
Welcoming Change

Menopause is not just a phase; it's a profound journey that every woman embarks on, marking the transition into what can be the most vibrant chapter of her life. It's a time of transformation, where the shifts within can spark a powerful metamorphosis. This initiation invites us to reimagine our lives, embracing change with grace and strength.

The spectrum of experiences during menopause is as diverse as the women it touches. Some navigate this journey with minimal turbulence, while others find themselves amidst a storm of physical and emotional changes. It's essential to acknowledge that no two journeys are the same, but every woman's experience is valid, important, and deserving of understanding and care.

Our society often paints menopause in a less-than-flattering light, framing it as something to be endured rather than celebrated. This narrative is not only outdated but profoundly inaccurate. Menopause is not a loss; it's a liberation - a journey towards self-discovery, empowerment, and a deeper connection with oneself.

With the right knowledge and support, you can navigate this transition with confidence and optimism. This begins by dispelling myths that surround menopause, providing you with accurate information to understand the changes happening within your body and mind. Knowledge is power, and with it, you can take charge of your menopause journey.

Recognising the early signs and symptoms of menopause is crucial. They serve as the body's way of signalling the onset of this new chapter. By tuning into these cues, you can start adapting your lifestyle, diet, and mindset early on, laying a strong foundation for the years to come.

Navigating through hot flushes, sleep disturbances, and emotional fluxes can be challenging. Yet, it's possible to mitigate these discomforts through a combination of medical knowledge, lifestyle adjustments, and holistic approaches. Every strategy you learn and apply is a step towards reclaiming your well-being and vibrance.

This journey isn't just physical; it's deeply emotional and psychological. Understanding and accepting the shifts in your emotional state and self-identity are pivotal. It's an opportunity to rebuild and reinforce your sense of self. Embracing change allows for profound personal growth and a renewed sense of purpose.

The spiritual dimension of menopause often goes unspoken. Yet, many women find this period a time for introspection and seeking deeper meaning in life. This transformative phase can lead to an awakening of sorts, where life's priorities are reassessed, and inner peace cultivated.

Nutrition and exercise play a key role in navigating menopause with vitality. A balanced diet and tailored exercise regime can dramatically alleviate symptoms, boost your energy, and improve your overall quality of life. This book will guide you in creating a lifestyle that supports you through menopause and beyond.

Further, alternative therapies and supplements offer additional avenues for relief and well-being. It's important to approach these with an informed mind, understanding their benefits and risks. Menopause is a holistic journey, and exploring various options allows you to construct a comprehensive self-care plan.

Medical treatments and considerations form another pillar of managing menopause effectively. Hormone Replacement Therapy (HRT) and other medical options can offer respite for many symptoms. Being well-informed about these helps you make choices that align with your health goals and personal beliefs.

Addressing cardiovascular health, bone integrity, and the genitourinary syndrome of menopause are crucial for long-term well-being. This stage of life calls for proactive steps towards preserving and enhancing your health, ensuring vitality in the years that follow.

The impact of menopause extends beyond the individual; it touches relationships, communication, and even the workplace. It's a time to articulate needs, set boundaries, and cultivate understanding with loved ones and colleagues alike. Effective communication and support networks are invaluable during this time.

Embracing creativity, hobbies, and financial planning not only enriches life but also bolsters mental health and provides a sense of security and fulfillment. These elements contribute to a wholesome approach towards menopause, one that champions joy, creativity, and financial independence.

As we embark on this journey together through the pages of this book, remember that menopause is not an end but a beginning. It's an invitation to embrace change with an open heart, to rewrite the script of what this stage of life represents. With knowledge, understanding, and a positive outlook, we can transform menopause into a period of renewal, empowerment, and joy. Welcome to your transformative journey.

Chapter 1:
Understanding Menopause

Transitioning into menopause marks a significant phase in a woman's life; it's a period brimming with change, challenging long-held notions about femininity and aging. This chapter serves as a foundational guide to comprehending the menopausal transition, shedding light on the biological symphony that orchestrates this phase. It aims to demystify menopause, disentangling facts from prevalent myths, and providing a clear-eyed view of what menopause is—and what it isn't. As we delve into this subject, it's crucial to remember that menopause is not merely an end to fertility, but a gateway to a new, vibrant chapter of life. By understanding the intricacies of hormonal shifts, we equip ourselves with the knowledge to navigate this transition more smoothly. It's an opportunity to reconnect with one's body, to listen and adapt, ensuring that we journey through menopause not with apprehension, but with confidence and a sense of empowerment. So, let's embark on this journey together, embracing the changes, and understanding that menopause, far from being a taboo or a decline, marks the beginning of a richly rewarding stage of life, flourishing with potential for transformation and growth.

The Biological Dance: Hormones in Transition

As we journey further into the heart of understanding menopause, it's paramount to cast our focus on the very essence of what triggers this transformative phase in a woman's life: the intricate ballet of hormones undergoing transition. This period, often surrounded by an aura of mystique and myriad misconceptions, is nothing short of a biological marvel, a testament to the resilience and adaptability of the female body.

At its core, menopause marks the cessation of menstruation, a sign that the ovaries have concluded their role in egg production. But this is not merely an on-off switch. It's a gradual, often complex process where the levels of estrogen and progesterone, the key players in a woman's reproductive system, begin to ebb and flow in a less predictable manner. This dance of hormones doesn't happen in isolation; it reverberates through the entirety of one's body, influencing a spectrum of physiological and psychological experiences.

Estrogen, often hailed as the quintessential female hormone, plays a critical role beyond fertility. Its decline is associated with various menopausal symptoms such as hot flushes, mood changes, and sleep disturbances. However, it's crucial to understand that these symptoms are merely transient, a natural part of the body finding its new equilibrium.

Progesterone's waning levels also contribute to the menopause symphony, primarily affecting menstrual patterns and contributing to the onset of perimenopause. The interplay between estrogen and progesterone is delicate, and as these hormones modulate, they signal the body to navigate through these changes.

It's worth noting that menopause is not a one-size-fits-all experience. The spectrum of hormonal changes is wide, and as such, each woman's journey is uniquely her own. These variations underscore the importance of understanding and embracing menopause not as a singular event but as a personalised experience.

Amidst these transitions, the role of other hormones, such as testosterone, shouldn't be overshadowed. While predominantly associated with male characteristics, testosterone plays a part in women's bone density, muscle strength, and sexual desire. Its subtle decline during menopause contributes further to the complex hormonal puzzle.

Understanding these hormonal shifts is empowering. It dismantles the fears and uncertainties that often shroud menopause, illuminating it instead as a natural, albeit significant, stage in a woman's life. Knowledge about these changes allows for a proactive approach to health and well-being during menopause.

Armed with awareness, it becomes possible to mitigate some of the discomforts associated with hormonal fluctuations. Lifestyle modifications, such as a balanced diet, regular physical activity, and stress reduction techniques, can significantly impact how one experiences menopause. These actions don't just address symptoms; they're a form of self-care, a dedication to navigating menopause with grace and strength.

Moreover, it's a period that underscores the importance of medical guidance and support. Engaging in open dialogues with healthcare professionals about hormone therapy options, alternative treatments, and strategies to manage symptoms is crucial. These conversations are part of the broader narrative of taking control of one's menopause journey.

However, it's essential to look beyond the immediate horizon of menopause symptoms and hormone transitions. This stage of life also opens the door to profound personal growth and introspection. It's a time when many women find a renewed sense of purpose, explore new interests, and forge stronger connections with their bodies and minds.

In embracing menopause, there's an opportunity to reframe the narrative around ageing and women's health. It's a chance to celebrate resilience and the beauty of transition, recognising that menopause is not an end but a new beginning. This perspective is not just uplifting; it's transformative.

The biological dance of hormones in transition is indeed intricate, but it's also a testament to the dynamism of life itself. With each change, there's potential for renewal and growth. Menopause, with all its complexities, is a compelling invitation to embark on a journey of self-discovery and empowerment.

As we navigate through the nuances of hormone transitions, let's remember that menopause is not merely a phase to endure but a stage to embrace with curiosity, compassion, and confidence. It's a chapter where the wisdom of the body and the strength of the spirit come together, guiding us towards a renewed sense of wellbeing and vitality.

In concluding this exploration of hormones in transition, it's clear that menopause is much more than a biological process. It's a holistic experience that encompasses physical, emotional, and spiritual dimensions. By approaching menopause with an informed and open heart, we can harness its transformative power and step into this new chapter with joy and pride.

Thus, the dance of hormones during menopause is not just a biological phenomenon. It's a journey of change, an opportunity for growth, and a celebration of womanhood. Let's embrace this dance, not as spectators but as active participants, ready to explore the richness and depth of this significant life stage.

Debunking Myths: What Menopause Is and Isn't

The journey through menopause is as unique as the individual experiencing it, yet it's often shrouded in mystery and misconception. As we traverse this path together, it's vital to dispel the myths that cloud our understanding and embrace the truths that empower us.

Menopause isn't merely a phase; it's a significant life transition that heralds a new era of personal growth and discovery.

A widespread myth is that menopause signals the end of femininity and sexuality. This couldn't be further from the truth. Menopause is not an extinguishing of the vibrant woman you are; rather, it's a rebirth. Your body is adapting, not diminishing. Sexuality and sensuality, far from waning, can find new depth and expression as you learn to navigate the changes within your body and embrace them with confidence and grace.

Another common misunderstanding is that menopause invariably leads to severe mood swings and emotional instability. While hormonal changes can affect mood, the extent and severity vary widely among women. It's not a one-size-fits-all experience. Recognizing and addressing these changes is a step towards managing them effectively, not surrendering to them as an inevitable plight.

Many believe that the onset of menopause means the end of physical vitality and the beginning of rapid decline. However, this period can also be the start of an invigorating chapter where women can focus more intensely on their health, exploring new fitness regimes and nutritional plans to fortify their bodies for the years ahead.

It's often thought that menopause is a solitary journey, one to be endured rather than shared. Yet, this transition provides an invaluable opportunity to connect with others, sharing experiences and strategies for managing symptoms. Far from isolating, menopause can broaden your social network and deepen existing relationships through shared understanding and support.

Some assert that menopause consists only of negative symptoms and experiences. While challenges certainly exist, this transition also ushers in positive changes. Many women report feeling a newfound sense of liberation and confidence, with a greater understanding of their bodies and needs.

There's also the myth that menopause can be completely controlled and managed through medication alone. Menopause is a complex interplay of physical, emotional, and psychological changes that require a holistic approach to management. Lifestyle adjustments, diet, exercise, and mental health support play crucial roles alongside medical treatments.

Another myth posits that menopause is a sharp, defined point in time. In reality, it's a gradual process with three stages: perimenopause, menopause itself, and postmenopause. Understanding these phases can help demystify the experience and prepare for the changes each phase brings.

The belief that menopause only affects women in their late 50s is another misconception. In truth, the symptoms can start much earlier, during the perimenopausal years. Every woman's timeline is different, and some may experience signs in their 40s or even earlier.

Contrary to the myth that life diminishes after menopause, many women report feeling more energized and purposeful. Freed from the concerns of menstruation and contraception, they find more space to explore new interests, careers, and personal development.

It's also incorrectly assumed that menopause invariably results in decreased libido. While some women may experience changes in sexual desire, others find a renewed or even heightened interest in sexual intimacy, unencumbered by previous constraints.

The myth that menopause is purely a women's issue is one that needs dispelling. The effects of menopause ripple out, touching partners, families, and friends. An open dialog about its impacts can lead to greater empathy and support from the wider community.

Another misconception is that menopause leads to inevitable weight gain. While hormonal changes can affect metabolism, weight control is still possible through healthy lifestyle choices. Understanding and adapting to your body's changing needs can help maintain a healthy weight.

Finally, the idea that menopause marks the beginning of a woman's twilight years is an outdated and disempowering myth. Many women view menopause as a new dawn, an opportunity to focus on themselves, their aspirations, and their well-being.

In debunking these myths, our goal isn't just to correct misinformation but to shift the narrative surrounding menopause. It's not a decline into obscurity; it's a step into a new, vibrant chapter of life, marked by wisdom, strength, and a deeper sense of self. With the right understanding, support, and approach, this stage can be one of the most empowering of your life.

Chapter 2:
Early Signs and Symptoms

As we transition from a comprehensive understanding of menopause in Chapter 1, it's pivotal to dive into the early signs and symptoms that herald this transformative phase. Recognising these early markers is not just about foreseeing change; it's about empowering yourself with knowledge to navigate this journey with confidence and grace. The prelude to menopause can be a subtle yet profound experience, encompassing both physical and emotional signals that signify your body's intricate biological dance. From the whispers of hot flushes that come without warning to the unexpected waves of emotional shifts, these signals beckon us to listen closely and respond with care. It's a period coloured by change, indeed, but understanding these signs equips us to ride the waves with resilience rather than being caught off guard. This chapter is not just about listing symptoms; it's about redefining them as signals, as a language your body uses to communicate its needs and its transitions. By tuning into this language, we can navigate these changes not as mere bystanders but as active participants in our health and well-being, shaping our journey through menopause to be as enriching and fulfilling as the chapters that preceded it.

Recognising the Prelude

In the grand symphony of your life, the menopause transition can be likened to an intricate prelude, hinting at the transformation ahead. It's a time when subtle, yet profound, changes begin to orchestrate within your body, signalling the onset of a new chapter. Recognising these early signs is paramount, as they serve as the body's gentle nudges towards awareness and adaptation. Whether it's a shift in your menstrual cycle, a sudden wave of warmth flushing through your body, or unexpected mood swings, these indicators are your body's way of communicating its evolving needs. By tuning into these changes, you're embarking on a journey not just of physical understanding but of self-discovery and empowerment. This section invites you to listen closely to your body's messages, decode its language, and take proactive steps towards embracing and managing the menopause transition with grace, knowledge, and confidence. Remember, recognising the prelude allows you to conduct your symphony with intention, harmonising your wellbeing with the upcoming waves of change.

Physical Indicators As we continue our journey through the tapestry of menopause, a critical chapter unfolds, revealing the physical signs that herald this transformative phase. It's paramount to recognise these indicators not as mere symptoms but as signposts guiding us through the intricate dance of change.

One of the most noticeable signs is the alteration in menstrual patterns. As you approach menopause, periods may become irregular - a signal from your body that the rhythm of your reproductive cycle is shifting. It's essential to approach these changes with a mindset of curiosity rather than concern, seeing them as natural steps in life's journey.

Hot flushes stand out as another hallmark of menopause, affecting a vast majority of women to varying degrees. These sudden waves of heat can sweep through your body without warning, leaving you seeking respite. Yet, within these moments of discomfort lies a profound reminder of your body's capacity to adapt and signal its needs.

Night sweats, closely related to hot flushes, can disrupt your sleep, leaving you yearning for a restful night. Rather than seeing it as an inconvenience, consider it as your body's way of communicating its transitional phase, encouraging you to seek solace and balance through calming practices.

The fluctuation of hormones may also lead to changes in skin and hair, manifesting as dryness or thinning. Embrace these changes by nurturing your body with the care and attention it deserves, transforming your daily skincare and haircare routines into acts of self-love and acceptance.

Vaginal dryness and discomfort, though often spoken about in hushed tones, warrant open conversation and care. They remind us of the importance of attending to all aspects of our health with kindness and openness, seeking support and solutions to embrace comfort once more.

Weight management becomes yet another area of focus during menopause. Hormonal shifts can affect metabolism, making it a prime time to explore new wellness practices, ensuring your approach to nutrition and exercise is aligned with your body's evolving needs.

The lessening density of bones, a silent change, calls for proactive steps towards strengthening bone health. It's a nudge to infuse your life with activities and nutrition that fortify your bones, embodying resilience and strength in every stride.

Joint and muscle discomfort might also nudge their way into awareness, urging you to explore gentle, strengthening exercises. Viewing these as opportunities for movement and connection with your body can transform discomfort into a path towards vitality.

Amidst these changes, an increase in urine frequency or urgency might be noticed, a reminder to nurture your pelvic floor health.

Viewing this as a call to engage with your body more deeply, you can discover strength and control in areas previously unattended.

Within this realm of change, some women experience heart palpitations, a fluttering reminder of the heart's capability to communicate the body's needs. Embracing this with calm and mindfulness can pave the way to understanding and nurturing your heart health.

This transition might also touch upon your sense of sight, with fluctuations leading to changes in vision. Seeing this as a metaphor for new ways of seeing yourself and the world can add a layer of depth to your journey through menopause.

Amidst the physical signs, breast tenderness may emerge as a tender reminder of your body's sensitivity to hormonal fluctuations. It invites you to treat your body with gentleness, understanding, and care, wrapping yourself in compassion.

As these physical indicators weave through your experience of menopause, remember, they're not mere symptoms to be eradicated but messages from your body. They call for attention, care, and perhaps most importantly, a rekindling of the relationship you have with your physical self. Embrace this dialogue with your body, seeing it as an opportunity for growth, transformation, and renewal.

By approaching these physical signs with a blend of curiosity, care, and compassion, you can navigate the waves of menopause not as a challenge to be overcome but as a passage to be embraced. It's a time to celebrate your body's wisdom, strength, and the incredible journey it's embarking upon. Let these physical indicators be your guide, a map to navigating menopause with grace, empowerment, and an enduring sense of wellbeing.

Emotional Signals As we delve further into the odyssey of menopause, it's pivotal to not only focus on the physical manifestations but to also confront and understand the emotional whirlwinds that often accompany this transition. Emotional signals during menopause are not just side effects; they are profound messengers, signalling changes within the body and mind, and reflecting the deep, internal processes at play.

It's common to experience a wide range of emotions during this stage, from ebbs of sadness to sudden surges of irritability. These feelings are not simply arbitrary but are closely linked to the hormonal shifts occurring within your body. Estrogen and progesterone, hormones that have been with you, steering your emotional ship since puberty, begin to fluctuate, and with them, your moods might too.

Understanding these emotional signals is not about taming them or boxing them into negativity. Instead, it's about acknowledging their presence, tracing their roots, and learning to navigate through them with compassion and patience. Many women report feelings of loss during this time, grieving for their youth or the fertility that was. It's entirely natural to feel this way, and important to allow yourself space to mourn.

Simultaneously, menopause can stir a pot of anxiety and stress. Questions about aging, attractiveness, and overall health can become more pronounced. Here, it's crucial to dissect these anxieties, to confront them with both the knowledge of menopause's natural course and an understanding of your value and beauty that transcends age.

Anger and irritability can also knock more frequently on your door. Small things that you may have brushed off previously now ignite a quicker fuse. Recognising this and implementing strategies such as mindfulness, breathing exercises, or even stepping away for a moment can be immensely beneficial. It's also helpful to communicate with those around you, sharing what you're going through. Most times, people want to help; they just need a window in.

Depression is another emotional signal that should not be ignored. While it's normal to have days dipped in blue, a persistent shadow of sadness requires attention. Here, the interplay between mindfulness, professional support, and possibly medication should be explored with care and guidance.

The flip side of this emotional rollercoaster can be periods of renewed energy and happiness. As you navigate through menopause, there will be moments where you feel a sense of liberation, unburdened from the worries of menstruation or contraception. Embrace these moments, let them refuel your journey through menopause, and remind you of the growth and wisdom being cultivated.

Aside from navigating these emotional signals for oneself, it's significant to understand how they might affect relationships. Patience can run thin, misunderstandings may crop up more easily, and therefore, clear, calm communication becomes paramount. Work on expressing your feelings without placing blame, and invite open dialogue.

A common yet less talked about emotional signal is a shift in libido. Changes in desire can stoke concerns about intimacy and relationships. Recognising this as a potential phase and finding new ways to connect emotionally and physically with your partner can usher in a deeper understanding and closeness.

Loneliness too can seep in, as you might feel that others can't quite grasp what you're going through. It's here that seeking out communities, whether through support groups, online forums, or even friends navigating the same waters, becomes invaluable. Sharing stories, frustrations, and victories can be immensely comforting and empowering.

Joy might seem like an elusive concept amid these tumultuous times, but it's there, nestled in the pauses and silences, waiting to be acknowledged. It's found in the strength you muster each day, the personal insights gained, and the sheer resilience displayed as you wade through these changes. Joy is there in the acceptance of this new phase of life, with all its challenges and triumphs.

While menopause might initially seem like a tumultuous storm to weather, with the right knowledge, tools, and attitudes, it can also be a period of profound personal growth and transformation. Understanding and tuning into your emotional signals is a critical step in this journey; they're not merely reactions to be quelled but voices to be heard, understood, and respected.

Treating yourself with kindness during this time is of utmost importance. Engaging in self-care activities, whether that's through nurturing hobbies, physical exercise, or simply time spent in nature, can provide a soothing balm for the emotional and physical shifts experienced.

Lastly, holding onto a vision of yourself beyond menopause, a vision filled with strength, wisdom, and vitality, can serve as a powerful anchor. Menopause is not the end of youth or femininity but rather a transition into a new, equally vibrant phase of life. Embrace it with grace, with courage, and most importantly, with an unwavering belief in yourself.

In conclusion, the emotional signals of menopause are myriad, complex, and deeply personal. They call for a journey inward, a navigation through the self, with all its nuances and colours. This chapter of your life, while challenging, holds the potential for immense personal discovery and growth. Let's walk through it together, with open hearts and minds, ready to embrace the myriad changes and emerge empowered and renewed.

Navigating the Waves of Change

As we venture deeper into the heart of menopause, understanding its early signs and symptoms becomes a beacon of insight, guiding us through this transitional voyage. It's a period marked not only by change but by transformation, an opportunity to embrace a new chapter with wisdom and grace. Yet, navigating through this phase can feel like sailing through uncharted waters, where each wave of change brings its own set of challenges and discoveries.

The journey through menopause is as diverse as the women who experience it. Some of us might notice subtle shifts in our bodies and minds, while for others, these changes can be more pronounced. Recognizing these signals early on serves as our compass, helping us to steer more effectively through the ups and downs, ensuring we're not merely surviving but thriving during this phase of our lives.

Physical indicators such as irregular periods or the infamous hot flushes are often the first signs that we're entering the perimenopausal waters. These changes are our body's way of signalling the beginning of a natural transition, spurred by the ebb and flow of our hormones. Yet, amidst these physical signs, there's a deeper, more nuanced layer to menopause, one that intertwines with our emotional and psychological realms.

Emotional signals, including mood swings and a noticeable shift in our mental well-being, are equally telling. They remind us that menopause isn't just a biological journey but a holistic one, affecting every facet of our being. It's in recognising these signs, both physical and emotional, that we gather the strength to navigate menopause with agency and intentionality.

Yet, acknowledging the changes is just the beginning. The real empowerment comes from understanding that these waves of change can be harnessed. Just as a skilled sailor uses the wind to propel her boat forward, we, too, can use our knowledge and strategies to glide more smoothly through menopausal waters. This involves a blend of self-care, informed choices about our health, and creating a support system that anchors us.

It's also crucial to debunk the myths surrounding menopause, many of which can cloud our perception of this stage of life. By arming ourselves with accurate information, we're better positioned to make choices that align with our personal health needs and lifestyles. This clarity not only illuminates our path but also empowers us to rewrite the narrative around menopause, viewing it not as an ending but as a powerful beginning.

Moreover, navigating the waves of change is about tuning into our bodies with compassion and curiosity. It's about listening deeply to the signals our bodies are sending and responding with care. Whether it's adapting our diet to support our changing nutritional needs, integrating exercise that feels rejuvenating, or exploring therapies that bring balance, it's these acts of self-care that become the rudder steering us through menopause.

The emotional voyage of menopause, too, presents an opportunity for profound growth. It's a time when many of us reevaluate our priorities, relationships, and the essence of what brings us joy and fulfilment. This introspection can unearth new passions, deepen connections, and inspire a renewed sense of purpose. Navigating these emotional currents with grace invites a deeper connection with our inner selves and with those around us.

As we sail through these changes, let's not overlook the power of community. Sharing our stories, challenges, and triumphs with others creates a collective strength that buoys us all. It's in these shared experiences that we find understanding, empathy, and encouragement. Building a support network, whether through friends, family, or support groups, casts a lifeline that can pull us through even the stormiest of seas.

Another vital aspect of navigating menopause is addressing our mental well-being. The fluctuations in hormones can impact our cognitive functions and emotional health. Recognizing and seeking support for these changes is not a sign of weakness but of profound strength. It's a declaration that our mental health is just as important as our physical health.

Moreover, this transitional period can also impact our relationships and intimate connections. As our bodies and emotions undergo transformation, so too might our needs and desires within our relationships. Open, honest communication becomes our compass, guiding us towards understanding and intimacy, even as we navigate through changes.

Let's also embrace the opportunity to rekindle or discover new passions and hobbies. Menopause can be a catalyst for exploring new interests or dedicating time to those we've previously set aside. These pursuits not only enrich our lives but can also serve as a therapeutic outlet, fostering a sense of achievement and satisfaction.

In dealing with the physical aspects of menopause, such as managing hot flushes or ensuring cardiovascular health, knowledge and proactive management are key. Understanding the options available, from lifestyle adjustments to medical treatments, allows us to make informed decisions that best support our health and well-being throughout menopause and beyond.

As we navigate the waves of change, remember that menopause is not just a phase to endure but a passage to empower. It's a time to honour our bodies, embrace our evolving selves, and celebrate the wisdom that comes with this life stage. With each wave we ride, we're not only navigating menopause; we're embracing a journey of transformation, growth, and renewal.

So, let us sail forth with confidence, supported by knowledge, embraced by community, and inspired by the boundless possibilities that lie ahead. Menopause is more than a biological transition; it's an invitation to rediscover ourselves, reframe our narratives, and revel in the depth of experience that this stage of life brings. Together, let's navigate these waves with courage, curiosity, and an open heart, ready to welcome the myriad of changes as gateways to empowerment and renewal.

Chapter 3:
The Physical Journey

As we delve into the heart of menopause, understanding the physical journey is crucial. This chapter serves as your map through the significant corporeal changes that accompany this transition. Navigating through hot flushes, changes in sleep patterns, weight fluctuation, and shifts in libido can feel like crossing unfamiliar terrain. Yet, it's important to view these changes not as obstacles but as segments of a path leading towards greater self-understanding and health. By embracing the knowledge presented here, you can arm yourself with the strategies necessary to manage these physical symptoms effectively. It's about more than seeking relief; it's about transforming your approach to your body and its needs during menopause. Each person's journey is unique, but the destination remains the same: finding peace and vitality in this new chapter of life. Rest assured, you're not merely surviving this physical journey; you're learning to thrive within it. Together, let's explore how to navigate these changes with grace, compassion for oneself, and a proactive mindset that turns challenges into opportunities for growth.

Navigating Through Hot Flushes

For many women, hot flushes are the hallmark of menopause, a sudden warmth that sweeps over the body, leaving one flushed and often perspiring. Understanding them isn't just about coping; it's about reclaiming a sense of control over your body during this transformative time. Hot flushes can feel like an unexpected guest, arriving without warning and disrupting your peace. Yet, within these moments of discomfort lies an opportunity to deepen our understanding and connection to our bodies.

Hot flushes vary widely in frequency and intensity, making them unpredictable. Some women may experience them a few times a week, while others might face them several times throughout the day. It's the body's response to the fluctuating levels of hormones, particularly oestrogen, as it adjusts to this new phase of life. Recognising this process as a normal physiological transition rather than an inconvenience can shift our perception and response to it.

The triggers of hot flushes can be as varied as the symptoms themselves. Common culprits include spicy foods, caffeine, stress, and even changes in the external environment like a warm room. Journaling your experiences and triggers can unveil patterns, empowering you to navigate through these moments with greater ease. Anticipating and avoiding known triggers is a proactive step towards reducing the frequency and severity of hot flushes.

Diet plays a crucial role in managing hot flushes. Foods rich in phytoestrogens, such as soy, flaxseeds, and certain nuts, can offer a natural avenue to balance hormones. Pairing a phytoestrogen-rich diet with regular hydration helps the body cool down more effectively during a hot flush. Consider it an act of nourishment, providing your body with what it needs to transition smoothly through menopause.

Exercise, too, contributes significantly to alleviating hot flushes. Engagement in regular, moderate activity, such as walking or yoga, can help regulate the body's internal thermostat. Studies suggest that women who maintain an active lifestyle report a reduction in the intensity and frequency of flushes. It's an invitation to reconnect with your body, to move with intent and mindfulness.

Breathing techniques offer an immediate remedy during a hot flush. Deep, controlled breathing can empower you to ride the wave of heat with composure. It's about harnessing the mind's capacity to influence the body, utilising breath as a bridge between the two. Practising mindfulness or meditation regularly can enhance this skill, providing a tool not only for managing hot flushes but for enriching your overall well-being.

Dress in layers to ensure that you can adjust your comfort level with the changing internal temperatures. Opting for natural, breathable fabrics can prevent heat from being trapped near the body, offering an easy, practical strategy to manage flushes. It's a simple adjustment that can make a substantial difference in your comfort throughout the day.

Hormone Replacement Therapy (HRT) is another avenue for those who experience severe hot flushes. Consulting with a healthcare professional to discuss HRT's benefits and risks can offer clarity. It's about making informed choices, recognising the array of options available to support you through menopause.

Alternative therapies, such as acupuncture and herbal remedies, have been known to offer relief for some women. While the scientific community is still exploring the complete efficacy of these treatments, personal testimonies suggest they could be worth considering. It underscores the importance of an open, exploratory mindset, willing to test different strategies to discover what works for you.

Staying connected with a supportive community, whether online or in person, can provide emotional comfort and practical advice. Sharing stories and solutions with others who are navigating similar experiences can be incredibly empowering. It's a reminder that you're not alone on this journey and that collective wisdom can light the way.

Educating those around you about what you're experiencing can foster empathy and understanding, creating a supportive environment at home and work. It underscores the importance of communication, of articulating your needs and boundaries. Knowledge is not only power for you but for those around you, enabling them to support you more effectively.

Finally, cultivating a positive mindset towards menopause and its symptoms can profoundly impact your experience. Viewing hot flushes and other symptoms as signs of a profound internal transformation allows you to navigate this journey with grace and resilience. It's about embracing menopause not as an end but as a new beginning, a gateway to a deeper understanding and appreciation of your body.

Remember, the journey through menopause is as unique as you are. While hot flushes might be a common thread, how you weave them into your life's tapestry is entirely up to you. Strategies and solutions abound, but the key lies in personalisation — finding what resonates with your body, lifestyle, and preferences.

In embracing and navigating through hot flushes, there resides a potent opportunity for growth and empowerment. Menopause is not merely a series of symptoms to be endured but a transition to be navigated with intention, understanding, and care. It's a time to turn inwards, to listen and respond to your body's needs, crafting a journey through menopause that is uniquely yours, marked by strength, wisdom, and wellbeing.

As we continue to explore the physical journey of menopause in the following sections, keep in mind the strategies and insights shared here. They're tools in your kit, designed to support and empower you through not just hot flushes, but all aspects of this transformative phase. Menopause, with all its challenges and changes, also brings with it a profound opportunity for renewal and growth. It's an invitation to redefine and rediscover yourself, to step into a phase of life marked by wisdom, strength, and a deepened sense of self.

Sleep and Menopause: Finding Rest Again

The journey through menopause is unique for every woman, characterised by a myriad of changes that can transform not just the body, but the spirit and the mind. Among the many adjustments, sleep disturbances stand out as particularly challenging for many. We embark on this chapter with a focus on navigating these nighttime disruptions and uncovering strategies to reclaim the restorative sleep that is so essential during this phase.

Why does menopause so often bring with it a struggle to maintain consistent, deep sleep? The answers lie in the symphony of hormonal changes. Oestrogen and progesterone, key conductors in this biological orchestra, don't just influence fertility and mood; they play critical roles in regulating sleep cycles. As their levels fluctuate and overall diminish, the delicate balance needed for seamless sleep can be upset, leading to insomnia or fragmented sleep patterns.

Hot flushes and night sweats are infamous companions of menopause, serving as abrupt awakenings that can shatter slumber. Imagine finally drifting off to sleep, only to be wrenched back to consciousness by an intense wave of heat - it's a scenario many menopausal women know all too well. The impact on sleep quality and overall wellbeing can be profound, leaving one feeling exhausted before the day even begins.

Yet, it's not all doom and gloom. With awareness and proactive management, restful nights can be within reach again. A cornerstone of this reclamation process involves establishing a sleep-conducive environment - a cool, quiet, and comfortable bedroom that invites relaxation and eases the body into sleep. Consider temperature-regulating beddings and sleepwear, designed to mitigate the discomforts of night sweats.

Another key strategy lies in embracing a consistent sleep routine. Going to bed and waking up at the same time every day, even on weekends, can significantly improve sleep quality. This regularity helps to anchor your body's internal clock, easing the transition to sleep and promoting a more uninterrupted night's rest.

Mindful of the stimulating effects of blue light from screens, it's wise to wind down with technology-free relaxation techniques in the evening. Whether it's through reading, meditation, or a soothing bath, finding your personal ritual to signal to your body that it's time to rest can make a world of difference.

Exercise, too, holds an invaluable place in the quest for better sleep during menopause. Regular physical activity, particularly in the morning or afternoon, can deepen sleep. However, it's important to avoid vigorous exercise close to bedtime, as this can invigorate the body, counteracting your efforts to relax.

Dietary considerations also play a pivotal role. Caffeine and alcohol, often culprits in disrupting sleep patterns, are best consumed in moderation and not close to bedtime. Lighter evening meals can fend off discomfort that might hinder sleep, and certain foods known for their sleep-promoting properties, such as almonds or chamomile tea, can be wonderful additions to your diet.

For those whose sleep issues persist despite lifestyle adjustments, it's important to explore other avenues. Cognitive behavioural therapy for insomnia (CBT-I) is a non-pharmaceutical approach that has proven effective for many, addressing the underlying thoughts and behaviours contributing to sleep disturbances.

Hormone replacement therapy (HRT) offers another avenue for relief, particularly for those whose sleep disturbances are tightly interwoven with hot flushes and night sweats. By easing these symptoms, HRT can indirectly nurture better sleep, though it's essential to thoroughly discuss the benefits and risks with a healthcare professional.

Let's not underestimate the power of support networks during this time. Sharing experiences and solutions with other women navigating similar challenges can not only provide practical advice but also a sense of solidarity and understanding. You're not alone on this journey, and sometimes, drawing strength from others' stories can illuminate your path to restful nights.

It's time to shift our perspective on sleep during menopause. Rather than viewing it as a battle to be fought, let's approach it as an opportunity for growth and adaptation. Recognising and embracing the changes in our bodies as they transition into this new phase, we can develop strategies and routines that honour and support our need for rest.

Remember, achieving restful sleep amid menopause is not an elusive dream. It requires patience, adaptation, and sometimes, professional guidance, but it is entirely possible. As women, we've navigated countless phases of change throughout our lives, harnessing our resilience and adaptability. Menopause, with all its challenges and transformations, is yet another chapter in our continuous journey of growth.

In reclaiming your night's rest, you reclaim your energy, your vitality, and your zest for life's next adventures. With each restful night, you're not just sleeping better; you're taking a bold step towards embracing menopause as a phase of empowerment and renewal. Let's celebrate this journey, for in its challenges lie opportunities to rediscover ourselves and forge a path of health and wellness that carries us forward with grace and strength.

Managing Weight and Metabolism

As we journey through the physical aspects of menopause within this chapter, it's crucial to shine a light on a concern that resonates deeply with many – managing weight and metabolism. The fluctuations in hormone levels experienced during this transformative period can significantly impact our body's ability to regulate weight and metabolise food efficiently.

Understanding the biological underpinnings is the first step towards empowerment. Menopause heralds a decrease in oestrogen levels, a hormone that's not only pivotal for reproductive functions but also plays a key role in managing lipid metabolism. This change can make maintaining a healthy weight more challenging but certainly not impossible.

Throwing restrictive diets out of the window, the focus should pivot towards nourishing your body with balanced, nutritious foods. Incorporating a variety of fruits, vegetables, whole grains, and lean proteins can support your metabolism and provide the nutrients your body craves during this time.

Hydration is another cornerstone of healthy weight management. Drinking enough water throughout the day supports metabolic function, aids in digestion, and helps you to feel fuller, potentially curbing unnecessary snacking.

Physical activity, while always important, becomes even more so during and after the menopause transition. Exercise isn't just a tool for weight management; it's a powerful means to enhance mood, improve sleep, and boost overall energy levels. Tailoring your exercise regime to include a mix of cardiovascular, strength-training, and flexibility exercises can address the body's evolving needs.

Stress management shouldn't be overlooked either. High-stress levels can lead to comfort eating and a slower metabolism. Practices such as yoga, meditation, and mindful breathing can mitigate stress, thereby indirectly supporting healthy weight management.

While dietary adjustments and increased physical activity are vital, acknowledging the importance of sleep is equally critical. Poor sleep can disrupt the body's hunger hormones, leading to increased appetite and weight gain. Endeavour to cultivate a calming bedtime routine and aim for seven to nine hours of quality sleep per night.

The concept of mindful eating can be transformative. It involves paying close attention to the experience of eating, savouring each bite, and listening to the body's hunger and fullness signals. This practice can prevent overeating and improve your relationship with food.

Consideration of portion sizes is a practical approach to managing weight. It's easy to overeat, even healthy foods, so being mindful of how much goes onto your plate is a simple yet effective strategy.

Remember, weight management during menopause isn't solely about the numbers on a scale. It's about embracing healthy habits that support your body's changing needs, enhancing your wellbeing, and feeling your best.

Seeking support can also make a significant difference. Whether it's consulting a nutritionist, joining a support group, or partnering with a friend on a similar journey, having encouragement and accountability can be incredibly motivating.

It's also crucial to strive for consistency rather than perfection. Small, sustainable changes to your lifestyle are more beneficial in the long run than drastic overhauls that are hard to maintain.

Listening to your body is perhaps one of the most profound pieces of advice. Each person's experience of menopause is unique, and what works for one may not work for another. Pay attention to how your body responds to different foods, types of exercise, and lifestyle changes, and adjust accordingly.

Lastly, it's important to approach weight and metabolism management with kindness and patience. Menopause is a significant life transition, and navigating its challenges requires time and self-compassion. Celebrate your successes, learn from setbacks, and always remember that you're not alone in this journey.

Maintaining a healthy weight and efficient metabolism during menopause is indeed achievable. By focusing on balanced nutrition, consistent physical activity, stress reduction, and self-compassion, you can support your body through this transformative time with grace and strength. Embrace this chapter of your life with an open heart and a commitment to self-care, and watch as you flourish in ways you never thought possible.

The Landscape of Libido

As we navigate through the myriad changes that menopause brings, it's essential to address an aspect often whispered about but rarely explored with depth and honesty: the landscape of libido during this pivotal time. Many women experience a shift in their sexual desire and function, which can be both confusing and distressing. Yet, this chapter is dedicated to shedding light on this sensitive area, empowering women to understand and embrace the changes, and, most importantly, to find joy and satisfaction in their intimate lives once again.

The fluctuation of hormones during menopause directly impacts libido. Estrogen and testosterone levels, which play crucial roles in female sexual desire and satisfaction, decrease, leading to changes in how arousal and pleasure are experienced. It's akin to the body's symphony playing a slightly different tune, one that requires us to listen more intently and learn to appreciate new rhythms and melodies.

One of the most noticeable changes may be in vaginal health. Reduced estrogen levels can lead to vaginal dryness, making sexual activity uncomfortable or even painful for some. This physical discomfort naturally affects desire, as the anticipation of pain dampens the emotional and physical longing for intimacy.

However, it's not all a tale of waning desire and discomfort. This time also offers an opportunity for exploration and rediscovery. Without the worry of pregnancy, menopause can be a time to explore new dimensions of your sexuality and intimate relationships. Communication with your partner becomes paramount. Expressing your feelings, desires, and the physical changes you're experiencing opens the door to a deeper understanding and connection.

Lubricants and moisturisers can play a significant role in enhancing comfort and pleasure during sex. They are not just practical aids but can be incorporated into lovemaking in a way that enhances intimacy. This is the time to experiment and find what works best for you, turning potential obstacles into opportunities for deeper exploration.

Creativity in your intimate life can lead to a rekindling of desire. Experimenting with new positions, practices, or even the time of day can bring a refreshing change. It's about finding what ignites that spark within you and embracing the journey of discovery with an open heart and mind.

For some, the dip in libido is closely tied to other menopausal symptoms such as sleep disturbances or mood swings. Addressing these accompanying symptoms holistically can indirectly benefit your sexual health. A good night's sleep or managing stress more effectively can do wonders for your libido. It's all about nurturing your wellbeing on all fronts.

Hormone replacement therapy (HRT) may be an option for some, offering relief from menopausal symptoms, including those affecting libido. It's crucial, however, to discuss this thoroughly with a healthcare provider, understanding the benefits and risks to make an informed decision that aligns with your personal health profile and preferences.

Exploring new forms of intimacy that don't necessarily involve intercourse can also be rewarding. Emotional closeness, sensual touch, and mutual massage can fulfil the human need for physical connection, reinforcing the bond with your partner in new and meaningful ways.

Regular exercise not only boosts your overall health but can also have a positive impact on your sex drive. Physical activity increases blood flow, enhances your mood, and boosts energy levels, all of which can contribute to a healthier libido. It's about feeling good in your body, embracing its strength and vitality.

Nutrition plays a role too. A balanced diet rich in essential nutrients can support your body's natural processes, including those related to sexual health. Foods that promote good circulation and heart health can also indirectly enhance libido by improving overall vitality and wellbeing.

It's important to approach this change with patience and kindness towards yourself. The journey through menopause is unique for every woman, and there is no 'right' way to experience or cope with changes in libido. What works for one may not work for another, and that's perfectly okay. It's about finding your own path, one that brings you joy, satisfaction, and a sense of wholeness.

Remember, intimacy is not merely a physical act but an emotional connection. This period of transition can deepen your understanding of your own needs, desires, and the ways in which you connect with your partner. It's an opportunity to redefine what intimacy means to you, embracing the changes with an open heart.

Finally, it's crucial to have open discussions with healthcare professionals about any concerns regarding libido and sexual health during menopause. There's a wealth of knowledge and support available, from medical treatments to lifestyle advice, all aimed at enhancing your quality of life during this time of transition.

The landscape of libido during menopause is indeed complex, but it's also filled with opportunities for growth, exploration, and deeper connection. With the right tools, knowledge, and support, this journey can be one of the most empowering experiences of your life, leading to a renewed sense of self and vitality in every aspect of your being.

Chapter 4:
Emotional Currents

The transition into menopause marks not just a physical transformation, but an emotional odyssey that can often catch us off guard. As we delve into the heart of understanding these emotional undercurrents, it's vital to recognise that the swings in our moods and mental states are not just figments of our imagination, but tangible shifts that deserve attention and care. With hormones ebbing and flowing like tides, feelings such as unexpected joy, sudden sadness, or unexplained irritability can become frequent visitors. However, instead of viewing these emotional fluctuations as adversaries, embracing them as part of this transformative phase can lead to a profound journey of self-discovery. Finding balance may sometimes feel like an elusive quest, yet it's within this very search that many women uncover strengths they didn't know they had. By employing strategies for emotional health, such as mindfulness, connection with supportive communities, and sometimes professional guidance, this chapter will explore how you can navigate these turbulent waters with resilience. Remember, amidst the tempest of change, there lies the opportunity to forge a more authentic and empowered self, ready to face the next chapter of life with grace and illumination.

Mood Swings and Mental Well-being

As we traverse the landscape of menopause, it's not just our physical selves that undergo transformation. Our internal world - our emotions, thoughts, and feelings - embarks on its own journey of change. Mood swings, a commonly experienced facet of this transition, can feel like being caught in an unpredictable current, where moments of tranquility are swiftly followed by turbulent waves of emotion. Understanding these emotional fluctuations is crucial for nurturing our mental well-being during this time.

The science behind mood swings in menopause is deeply rooted in the hormonal adjustments our bodies are making. As estrogen and progesterone levels fluctuate, so too does our brain's chemistry, particularly in how it handles neurotransmitters responsible for mood regulation. This can lead to feelings of sadness, irritability, or sudden joy. Recognizing that these swings are a natural part of the menopause journey can help us frame our experiences with kindness and patience.

Yet, it's not just about weathering the storm. It's about adapting our sails to navigate these emotional currents with grace. Simple lifestyle adjustments - such as integrating regular physical activity, ensuring a nutrient-rich diet, and prioritizing restful sleep - can significantly mitigate mood volatility. Each of these actions supports our body's hormonal balance and provides a sturdy foundation for emotional resilience.

Moreover, engaging in mindfulness practices such as meditation or deep-breathing exercises can be profoundly beneficial. These practices don't just offer a temporary haven of tranquility; they rewire our brain to better manage stress and anxiety, enhancing our overall mood stability. They remind us that amidst the chaos, there lies a center of calm we can return to.

It's also essential to remember that you're not alone on this journey. Connecting with others who understand what you're going through can be incredibly affirming. Whether it's joining a support group, participating in online forums, or just having a candid chat with friends going through similar experiences, sharing our stories can lighten our emotional load and foster a sense of community.

For some, the emotional upheavals of menopause may illuminate underlying mental health struggles that have been simmering beneath the surface. It's important not to brush these feelings aside as merely "part of menopause". Seeking professional support from therapists or counselors who specialize in menopause can provide the strategies and understanding needed to navigate these waters with care and compassion.

Self-care takes on a monumental importance during this time. It's not selfish; it's necessary. Crafting a personal self-care routine that includes activities you love, moments of solitude, and self-reflection, can reinforce your sense of self and provide an anchor in the midst of emotional fluctuations. Remember, caring for your mental well-being is just as important as attending to your physical health.

Journaling can also serve as a powerful tool in managing mood swings. Writing down your thoughts and feelings helps in processing emotions, identifying patterns, and reflecting on growth. It's a personal space for unfiltered expression, offering insights into our inner world and helping us navigate our emotional landscape with greater clarity.

Exploring creative outlets such as painting, writing, or gardening can catalyze emotional expression and offer therapeutic release. Engaging in creative activities has been shown to reduce stress, improve mood, and provide a sense of accomplishment and joy. It's an invitation to express ourselves in ways words cannot, turning our emotional currents into art.

Adopting a positive mindset towards menopause as a phase of growth and rebirth can also transform our experience. Instead of viewing mood swings and other symptoms as burdens, we can see them as indicators of change and evolution. This perspective shift can help us approach our experiences with curiosity and openness, seeking lessons and opportunities for personal development.

Learning to set boundaries is another essential skill during this time. Knowing when to say no, taking breaks when needed, and prioritizing your well-being helps in managing stress and maintaining emotional equilibrium. It's about honoring your needs and giving yourself permission to step back and rest.

Nutritional choices also play a key role in mental well-being. Incorporating foods rich in omega-3 fatty acids, antioxidants, and phytoestrogens can support brain health and mood regulation. Similarly, staying hydrated and limiting intake of alcohol and caffeine can help stabilize emotional fluctuations.

Laughter, often regarded as the best medicine, holds particular truth during menopause. Seeking moments of joy, humor, and lightness can uplift our spirits and provide a natural buffer against mood swings. It's about finding joy in the small things and allowing ourselves to embrace happiness amidst the chaos.

Lastly, practicing gratitude can shift our focus from the challenges of menopause to the abundance present in our lives. Taking time each day to acknowledge the things we are thankful for fosters positive emotions, reduces stress, and enhances our overall sense of well-being. It's a reminder of the beauty and strength within us and around us, guiding us gently through the waves of change.

In closing, mood swings during menopause are not merely obstacles to be endured but opportunities for profound personal growth and self-discovery. By nurturing our mental well-being with knowledge, care, and compassion, we can transform this journey into one of empowerment and renewal. Embrace the changes, for they are the keys to unlocking an even more vibrant and resilient version of yourself.

Finding Balance: Strategies for Emotional Health

Navigating the emotional currents of menopause requires not just understanding, but a toolbox of strategies designed to maintain emotional health. It's a stage that calls for a robust blend of self-care, support, and personal insight. As you step forward, remember, achieving balance doesn't mean avoiding emotions but learning how to navigate through them with grace.

One of the first steps in finding balance is recognising the emotional signals that your body is sending. These might come as mood swings, sudden tears, or perhaps unexplained irritability. It's not just your body that's in transition; your emotions are on a journey, too. Acknowledging these feelings as valid experiences can be incredibly freeing. It's okay to not feel okay all the time.

Another crucial strategy is building a support network. This could mean turning to friends who are at a similar stage in their lives, joining support groups, or even seeking professional guidance from a therapist who understands the nuances of menopause. Talking about your experiences, frustrations, and fears can lighten your emotional load and offer perspectives that you might not have considered.

Regular physical activity is a pillar for maintaining emotional equilibrium. Exercise isn't just good for your body; it's a powerful tool for mental health. It helps to alleviate stress, improve your mood, and can significantly boost your self-esteem. You don't need to run marathons—find an activity you enjoy and incorporate it into your daily routine.

Incorporating mindfulness and meditation into your day can also offer a sanctuary from the storm. These practices encourage you to live in the present moment and cultivate a deeper awareness of your thoughts and feelings without judgment. Even just a few minutes a day can make a considerable difference in how you navigate your emotional landscape.

Diet also plays a more significant role in emotional health than many realise. Nutrient-rich foods fuel both your body and mind. Eating a balanced diet can help stabilise mood swings and mitigate some of the emotional turbulence that can come with menopause. Paying attention to what, and when, you eat can be transformative.

Don't underestimate the power of sleep in the quest for emotional balance. Hormonal changes can wreak havoc on sleep patterns, but prioritising good sleep hygiene can make a difference. Aim for a serene sleep environment and a consistent bedtime routine to enhance your quality of sleep, which in turn, can improve emotional resilience.

Engaging in creativity is another avenue to explore for emotional health. Whether it's painting, writing, gardening, or any other creative outlet, these activities can offer a sense of accomplishment and joy. Creative pursuits not only serve as a stress reliever but can also be a form of self-expression and personal discovery.

Learning new skills or taking up hobbies isn't just about keeping busy; it's about keeping the mind engaged and stimulated. Continuous learning can build confidence and a sense of achievement, which are critical during a stage of life that might otherwise feel destabilising.

It's also important to cultivate gratitude. Keeping a gratitude journal or simply reflecting on positive aspects of your life can shift your focus from what's lacking to what's abundant. This practice has been shown to improve mental health and overall well-being by fostering a positive mindset.

Journeying through menopause, it's vital to set boundaries—both with others and with yourself. Learning to say no is not selfish; it's a necessary aspect of self-care. Establishing healthy boundaries allows you to conserve your energy for activities and people that nourish you.

Humour, too, can be a potent tool. Finding ways to laugh at the absurdities can lighten dark moments and bring relief. It's a way to bring lightness into your life, even when things feel heavy.

Forging a connection with nature has a grounding effect that can be incredibly balancing for emotional health. Whether it's a walk in the park, tending to a garden, or simply sitting by a window and observing nature, these moments can offer peace and a sense of connectedness to the world.

The strategy of embracing change rather than resisting it can be liberating. Viewing menopause as a transition into a new phase of life with its own opportunities and wisdom can transform the journey into one of growth and empowerment. It's not an end, but a beginning.

Ultimately, finding balance is a deeply personal journey that involves a tapestry of strategies. What works for one person may not work for another, and that's perfectly okay. It's about listening to your body, honouring your emotions, and taking daily steps towards wellness. Embrace this transformative stage with an open heart and mind, and remember, you're not alone. This journey is a shared one, and together, we can navigate the currents of change with strength and grace.

Chapter 5:
The Psychological Passage

The journey through menopause is as much a psychological passage as it is physical. This stage, pivotal and potent, commands a profound re-acquaintance with oneself, challenging and reshaping one's self-identity and body image. It's during this time that embracing change doesn't just mean coming to terms with the physical evolutions occurring within, but also confronting and accepting alterations in how we perceive ourselves and how we believe others perceive us. Amid fluctuating hormones and the myriad changes they instigate, the path to self-acceptance is both necessary and rewarding. It becomes crucial to navigate this passage with patience and kindness towards oneself, understanding that this transition is not merely a series of symptoms to be managed but an opportunity for profound personal growth and transformation. In recognizing and embracing this, one can find solace in the shared experiences of countless women before, finding strength in vulnerability and unity in individuality. The psychological journey through menopause, then, becomes not just about coping but about thriving, fostering a deeper, more compassionate relationship with oneself that paves the way for a future rich in possibility and suffused with a renewed sense of self-assurance and clarity.

Self-Identity and Body Image

As we manoeuvre through the web of menopause, one of the most profound transformations isn't just physical—it's deeply psychological. Amidst this shift, our perceptions of self-identity and body image come to the forefront, challenging us to reassess and rediscover who we truly are. This journey, while daunting, offers a unique opportunity to redefine our sense of self and embrace our changing bodies with kindness and grace.

Often, discussions around menopause focus on the tangible signs and symptoms, sidelining the significant impact it exerts on our self-perception and esteem. The mirror seems to reflect a stranger, leading to a disconnect between how we feel and how we see ourselves. Yet, it's essential to realise this isn't just a phase of loss but a stage of profound reinvention.

The fluctuations in our hormone levels play more than just a biological role; they touch upon the very essence of what it means to be us. Our body's changing shape and function can feel like a betrayal for some, making it crucial to navigate these waters with empathy towards oneself. To journey through menopause with strength, we must anchor our self-worth not in fleeting attributes but in the depth and richness of our experiences and achievements.

Reconstructing our body image doesn't happen overnight. It's a gradual process that begins with dispelling the societal myths that equate youth with beauty and worth. Menopause, rather than signalling an end, marks a transition into a phase of life ripe with potential, wisdom, and a different kind of beauty—one that's defined by character, resilience, and authenticity.

Comparing ourselves to our younger selves or others around us is a trap that only breeds dissatisfaction and discontent. Instead, celebrating our bodies for what they can do now, not just what they used to look like or be capable of, fosters a healthier self-image and appreciation for the present.

To aid in this transformation, mindfulness and self-compassion emerge as powerful tools. Practising mindfulness helps us remain grounded in the present moment, appreciating our bodies for the life they enable us to live. Meanwhile, self-compassion encourages a kinder internal dialogue, reminding us that we're not alone in our struggles and that perfection is an unrealistic and unattainable goal.

The media and popular culture often portray a skewed image of ageing, one that's either feared or ignored. It's imperative to seek out and create a new narrative—one that celebrates ageing as a natural and inevitable part of life, which brings with it a unique beauty and strength. Surrounding ourselves with positive role models and stories of women who've navigated this passage with grace can inspire and motivate us to do the same.

Body positivity during menopause also involves taking proactive steps towards self-care. Whether it's through nourishing our bodies with healthy foods, engaging in physical activities that bring joy, or dressing in ways that make us feel confident and comfortable, these actions empower us to reclaim our sense of agency over our bodies and our lives.

Let us not forget the power of communication. Sharing our experiences and feelings with friends, family, or support groups can not only provide comfort and solace but also normalise the conversation around menopause and body image. It's through these shared stories and collective wisdom that we can dismantle the stigma and build a more inclusive understanding of womanhood in all its stages.

Furthermore, exploring new interests and hobbies can act as a catalyst for discovering aspects of our identity that were previously overshadowed or unexplored. Menopause can thus become a gateway to new passions, friendships, and avenues for personal growth.

Embracing our evolving identity and body image during menopause also means acknowledging and honouring the journey it took to get here. Each wrinkle, grey hair, and change in our bodies tells a story of resilience, love, hardship, and triumph. These marks are not flaws to be hidden but badges of honour to be proudly displayed.

In essence, the menopause transition is as much about redefining our relationship with ourselves as it is about navigating the physical changes. It's an invitation to shed outdated beliefs and unattainable standards, offering instead a chance to embrace our authentic selves with unconditional love and respect.

Consider this passage as a call to action—a declaration that it's time to redefine what it means to age and to do so on our own terms. Let's collectively pave the way for a future where menopause is not dreaded but welcomed as a meaningful and empowering phase of life.

So, let us approach this chapter not merely as an end but as a vital turning point. With awareness, compassion, and courage, we can transform our experience of menopause from one of uncertainty and struggle to one of liberation and fulfilment. It's in our power to rewrite the narrative of ageing and, in doing so, empower not just ourselves but generations of women to come.

In closing, remember that menopause is not just a phase to endure but a journey to embrace. It's a time to celebrate the wisdom gained, the battles fought, and the beauty of evolving. Let's navigate this passage with grace, honouring our bodies and ourselves, for they've carried us this far and deserve nothing less than our deepest respect and love.

Embracing Change: The Path to Self-Acceptance

Approaching menopause is like standing at the threshold of a new era in one's life. It's a period marked not just by hormonal shifts but also by profound transformations in self-identity and body image. The journey towards self-acceptance during this phase is both challenging and enlightening. Here, we delve into strategies and mindsets that support embracing change wholeheartedly, leading to a deeper acceptance of oneself.

The sensation of change initiates a myriad of responses. Initially, it might seem daunting. You might look in the mirror and notice the first signs of menopause. It's a natural instinct to scrutinise these changes, sometimes with unease or frustration. Yet, it's vital to remember that these transformations are not just physical. They signal a new stage of empowerment and wisdom.

Self-acceptance begins with acknowledging these changes without judgement. It's helpful to view menopause not as an end but as a beginning. It represents an opportunity to reconnect with oneself on a more profound level. This period offers a chance to reassess your wants, needs, and aspirations in life from a place of experience and maturity.

The societal portrayal of menopause often leans towards the negative, presenting it as a phase to endure rather than celebrate. Challenge these narratives by seeking out positive stories and experiences. Your perspective plays a crucial role in shaping your menopause journey. By focusing on the positives, you encourage an environment of acceptance and growth.

Embracing change involves nurturing your mental and emotional well-being. Menopause can trigger a range of emotions, from vulnerability to resilience. Acknowledge these feelings as valid parts of the experience. Giving yourself permission to feel them fully is a step towards acceptance.

Practical steps towards self-acceptance include mindful practices such as meditation and journaling. These activities encourage introspection and self-compassion, enabling you to navigate your thoughts and emotions with grace. Moreover, they offer a safe space to explore your evolving identity.

Body image is a significant aspect of self-acceptance during menopause. As your body undergoes changes, it's crucial to cultivate a loving relationship with it. This can be achieved through practices that celebrate your body, such as engaging in physical activities that bring you joy and dressing in ways that make you feel confident and comfortable.

The power of community cannot be understated in this journey. Sharing your experiences with others who are navigating similar paths fosters a sense of belonging and support. It's comforting to realise you're not alone in your experiences. Listening to others can also provide new perspectives and strategies for embracing change.

Setting realistic expectations is another key aspect. Menopause is a natural life stage, and like any significant life event, it comes with its share of challenges and triumphs. Embracing this fact allows you to approach the journey with patience and understanding towards yourself.

Education about the physiological aspects of menopause equips you with knowledge, demystifying the process and reducing anxiety. Understanding the why behind the changes helps in adopting a more accepting attitude towards them.

Recognising the strengths acquired through life and how they can serve you during menopause is empowering. Your resilience, wisdom, and experience are invaluable assets. They not only assist in navigating this phase but also in rediscovering aspects of yourself that you may have overlooked.

Gratitude plays a pivotal role in the path to self-acceptance. By focusing on the aspects of life you're thankful for, you cultivate a positive mindset that supports well-being and acceptance. Gratitude for the journey thus far and the journey to come can be a powerful catalyst for growth and acceptance.

The relationship with oneself is often defined by internal dialogues. Pay attention to these conversations and strive to make them more compassionate and supportive. Remind yourself of your worth and achievements, encouraging a shift towards self-acknowledgement and acceptance.

Finally, embracing change and the path to self-acceptance is an ongoing process. It's not a destination reached overnight but a journey of continual growth and discovery. Celebrate each step forward, no matter how small, and be kind to yourself through setbacks.

Menopause, with all its complexities, is a remarkable journey of transformation. Embracing this change leads not just to self-acceptance but also to a renewed sense of vitality and purpose. It's an opportunity to reforge a relationship with oneself that's rooted in love, respect, and appreciation. Trust in your ability to navigate this path, and you'll find that menopause is not just about enduring change, but thriving through it.

Chapter 6:
The Spiritual Dimension

The journey through menopause is much more than a physical or emotional transition; it's a profound spiritual passage that invites us to explore the deeper layers of our being. In this chapter, we delve into how this period can become a pivotal moment for personal growth and spiritual awakening. Menopause isn't just about the end of a woman's reproductive years but also a time for reflection, self-discovery, and an opportunity to align more closely with one's authentic self. It's a phase where the noise of societal expectations can be silenced, allowing the inner voice of wisdom to emerge more clearly. Through engaging stories and practical advice, we'll explore how embracing this spiritual dimension can lead to a sense of inner peace and a deeper connection to the universe. Whether it's through meditation, mindfulness, or reconnecting with nature, we will uncover how these practices can complement traditional approaches to managing menopause symptoms, offering a holistic path to not just coping, but thriving. By acknowledging this spiritual journey, women are empowered to find meaning in transition, transforming what may initially appear as a daunting period into a celebration of a new phase of life that's ripe with potential for rediscovery and renewal.

Finding Meaning in Transition

As women, our journey through life is punctuated by a series of transitions, each carrying its own set of challenges and opportunities. Menopause is undoubtedly one of these significant transitions, marking not an end but rather a profound beginning. It's a time ripe for reflection, growth, and the cultivation of a deeper spiritual understanding of ourselves and our place in the cycle of life.

Many approach menopause with trepidation, focusing solely on its physical manifestations and the ways in which it signifies ageing. However, this perspective only scratches the surface of what is a much richer, more complex transition. Menopause is not just a series of biological changes, but a window to a spiritual awakening, where the search for meaning can bring about a transformation as significant on the inside as the changes happening on the outside.

Within every woman's experience of menopause, there lies an invitation to embark on a journey of self-discovery. This period prompts us to question and reassess who we are, what we value, and how we relate to the world around us. It's a time when the noise of fertility and the demands of others can quieten, allowing us to listen more intently to our own inner voice, guiding us towards a renewed sense of purpose and identity.

The key to finding meaning in this transition lies in embracing it with openness and curiosity. Instead of viewing menopause as a list of symptoms to be fixed, we can see it as a puzzle to be solved, a labyrinth with twists and turns that lead us deeper into understanding. It's an opportunity to learn, to grow, and to emerge more resilient and aware of our personal power and autonomy.

Spirituality during this phase can take many forms, none more valid than the other. For some, it may involve a reconnection with nature and the cycles that govern all life. For others, it might mean a deeper exploration of a faith tradition or the pursuit of practices like meditation and mindfulness that foster a sense of inner peace and connectedness.

It's also a time for healing old wounds and forgiving past grievances, both towards ourselves and others. Menopause can surface unresolved emotions and memories, but with this also comes the chance to release them, to find peace and to move forward with a lighter spirit.

The transition can significantly impact how we relate to our loved ones. It might challenge us to set healthier boundaries, communicate our needs more effectively, and deepen our connections by exploring new levels of honesty and vulnerability. Through these shifts, our relationships can become more meaningful and fulfilling.

Moreover, this phase of life invites us to contemplate our legacy - what we wish to leave behind and how we want to be remembered. It inspires us to contribute, to mentor, and to share the wisdom we've accumulated. Our experiences, trials, and triumphs hold the power to inspire and guide those who follow in our footsteps.

Employing creativity as a spiritual practice can be particularly enriching during menopause. Engaging in creative activities, whether it's writing, painting, gardening, or any form of artistic expression, can bring solace and joy. It allows us to express ourselves in ways that words sometimes can't, tapping into deep, untouched parts of our being, and facilitating a form of healing.

Physical activity too can be a spiritual endeavor. Through movement, whether it's yoga, dance, or walking in nature, we can find a profound sense of connection to our bodies, to the earth, and the rhythm of life. This embodied practice can help ease not just the physical but also the emotional and spiritual symptoms of menopause, reminding us of our strength and resilience.

Nutrition is another area where the spiritual intertwines with the physical. Menopause can encourage us to nurture our bodies with intention, choosing foods that not only nourish us but also connect us to the earth and our community. This mindful approach to eating can become a spiritual practice in its own right, one that honors the body as a temple and food as a sacred gift.

It's important to remember, however, that finding meaning in transition is not a linear process. It's marked by ups and downs, moments of clarity followed by periods of confusion. But even in the struggle, there is growth. Each step, no matter how faltering, is a step towards becoming more authentically ourselves, more aligned with our values and our soul's purpose.

Support from a community of like-minded individuals can be invaluable on this journey. Sharing stories and experiences can lighten our load, offer new perspectives, and remind us that we're not alone. Together, we can navigate the challenges and celebrate the triumphs, forging a path filled with compassion, understanding, and solidarity.

In the end, finding meaning in the transition of menopause is about recognizing and embracing the multitude of changes it brings - not just the end of fertility, but the beginning of a new era of freedom, wisdom, and introspection. It's a time to redefine what it means to be vibrant, vital, and alive, laying the groundwork for a future marked by joy, purpose, and deep fulfillment.

As we move through this transformative phase, let us hold onto the notion that menopause is not just a series of obstacles to overcome, but a gateway to a more profound understanding of ourselves and the world. It's an invitation to embark on the most important journey of all - the journey inward. And what we discover along the way can illuminate not just our own path but also the paths of those who walk beside us and after us.

Cultivating Inner Peace

As we venture further into the spiritual dimension of menopause, it becomes increasingly vital to discuss the cultivation of inner peace. This stage of life, often misunderstood and overlooked, holds the potential for profound spiritual awakening and growth. The key lies in embracing this period not as an end but as a vibrant chapter of reinvention and self-discovery.

Inner peace, often perceived as a serene state of mind unaffected by external disturbances, is much more attainable during menopause than one might initially think. It involves a harmony between the mind, body, and spirit, achieved through mindful practices and reflection. In this transformative phase, you're invited to delve into the depths of your being, exploring and confronting the myriad of emotions and changes with both grace and strength.

Commencing this journey requires a conscious decision to nurture your mental and emotional well-being. Meditation stands out as a beacon of tranquillity, guiding you towards inner peace. It's a practice that transcends mere relaxation, offering a pathway to understanding the fluctuations of your mind and, ultimately, to steadying them. Engaging in meditation daily can illuminate the shifts within and around you, encouraging a response rooted in calmness rather than reactive turmoil.

Similarly, the art of gratitude plays a crucial role in sculpting your inner landscape. Amidst the ebb and flow of menopausal symptoms, cultivating a mindset of thankfulness can significantly alter your perception. By appreciating the simple joys and acknowledging the lessons behind each challenge, a sense of inner peace gradually becomes ingrained in your daily life.

Another pillar supporting the temple of peace is mindfulness. This practice, focusing on present-moment awareness, gently steers you away from the regrets of the past and the anxieties of the future. It fosters a profound connection with the here and now, recognizing that each moment, no matter how trivial it seems, is a step on the journey of self-discovery and acceptance during menopause.

Integration of nature into your life also heralds a unique form of peace. The natural world, with its cycles and rhythms, mirrors the transitions you're experiencing. Spending time outdoors, whether it's tending to a garden or simply walking in a park, can recalibrate your spirit and remind you of the continuity present in all forms of life, including your own.

Physical well-being, though often categorised under a different heading, is inseparable from the quest for inner peace. A body nurtured by gentle, consistent exercise and nourished by wholesome foods sends ripples of comfort and satisfaction through the mind and spirit. This holistic approach ensures that the temple of your being is honoured and cared for in its entirety.

Journaling emerges as a powerful tool for self-reflection and emotional release. By documenting your thoughts, feelings, and experiences, you create a space for personal insight and clarity. This practice can be particularly therapeutic during menopause, a time when your internal world may feel more turbulent than usual.

Community, too, has a profound impact on your inner serenity. Connecting with others who are navigating similar paths fosters a sense of belonging and understanding. Sharing stories and strategies not only dispels feelings of isolation but also enriches your journey with diverse perspectives and support.

Forgiveness, both of self and others, unveils a pathway to peace that often goes unnoticed. Letting go of harboured grievances and self-criticism clears the way for compassion and self-acceptance, vital components of inner peace. It's about acknowledging your human imperfections and choosing to love yourself regardless.

Lastly, the concept of letting go stands as a liberating force. Menopause is an excellent teacher of this principle, prompting you to release outdated self-concepts, unhelpful habits, and anything else that no longer serves your highest good. Embracing this flux can transform fear into excitement for what lies ahead.

Cultivating inner peace during menopause is undeniably a personal and unique journey. Yet, it's also universal in its necessity. By committing to practices that resonate with your essence, you pave a path filled with wisdom, tranquillity, and profound understanding. Remember, this chapter of your life is an extraordinary opportunity for growth, a chance to flourish in ways previously unimaginable.

As this voyage unfolds, consider inner peace not as a distant dream but as a lived reality. With each step, with every breath, you have the power to nurture this serene state of being. The transformation menopause brings isn't just about physical changes—it's a spiritual awakening, inviting you to explore the depths of your soul and the boundless peace that resides within.

In summary, the cultivation of inner peace during menopause is an integrated process that involves attention to the mind, body, and spirit. Through practices such as meditation, gratitude, mindfulness, and fostering connections, you can navigate this period with grace and emerge with a profound sense of tranquillity and strength. Let this be a time of beautiful transformation, a period in life where you rediscover yourself and uncover the peace that has always been at the core of your being.

The journey is yours to embark upon, with each step an invitation to deeper understanding and peace. Embrace this sacred time with an open heart and mind, and let the quest for inner peace illuminate the path to a fulfilling and harmonious menopause experience.

Chapter 7:
Nutritional Foundations for Menopause

Navigating through menopause requires a holistic approach, where nutrition plays a pivotal role in managing symptoms and enhancing overall well-being. In this chapter, we'll delve into the essence of creating a balanced diet that's rich in essential nutrients, tailored specifically to the needs of women undergoing this transformative phase. Understandably, the body's requirements shift during menopause, emphasising the need for certain vitamins and minerals to support hormonal balance, bone density, heart health, and emotional stability. By prioritising nutrient-dense foods, integrating sources of calcium, magnesium, vitamin D, and phytoestrogens, and maintaining hydration, women can establish a strong nutritional foundation. Moreover, this chapter aims to demystify how dietary choices can either alleviate or aggravate menopausal symptoms, empowering women to make informed decisions that foster a sense of vitality and harmony. Alongside practical advice, we'll explore how embracing these nutritional principles can not only address the physical aspects of menopause but also uplift spirits and reinforce a positive, transformative journey towards embracing this new chapter with confidence and self-love.

Essential Nutrients and Menopause

Navigating the changes of menopause requires not just emotional resilience but also a mindful approach to nutrition. The relationship between what we eat and how we feel during this transformative phase can't be overstated. Like intricate dance partners, essential nutrients play a pivotal role in managing menopausal symptoms and ensuring a smoother transition.

Firstly, calcium is paramount. With the onset of menopause, the risk of osteoporosis spikes, making calcium-rich diets essential. This isn't merely about drinking more milk; it's about embracing a variety of calcium sources such as almonds, leafy greens, and fortified foods, ensuring your bones receive the support they need.

Similarly, vitamin D steps into the spotlight. Often dubbed the 'sunshine vitamin', it works hand in hand with calcium to fortify our bones. Yet, its benefits extend beyond that, possibly easing some menopausal symptoms and bolstering mood. Whether it's through brief daily sun exposure or dietary sources like oily fish and eggs, ensuring adequate vitamin D intake is crucial.

The significance of magnesium during menopause cannot be overlooked either. Known for its relaxation properties, it may help manage sleep issues and mood swings. Incorporating magnesium-rich foods like nuts, seeds, and whole grains into your diet can make a significant difference.

Omega-3 fatty acids, found abundantly in fish such as salmon, mackerel, and sardines, are celebrated for their anti-inflammatory properties. They're not just good for your heart; there's growing evidence that they can alleviate some menopausal symptoms such as hot flashes and depressive states.

Don't forget about fiber. Aside from its well-known digestive benefits, fiber helps regulate blood sugar levels, which can be particularly beneficial as menopause can alter your body's insulin sensitivity. Foods like fruits, vegetables, and whole grains are excellent fiber sources.

Equally important are antioxidants. These powerful substances combat oxidative stress and inflammation, which are notable adversaries during menopause. Brightly coloured fruits and vegetables are not only a feast for the eyes but are rich in antioxidants, offering an array of health benefits.

Water is another non-negotiable element. Staying hydrated helps combat the drying effects menopause can have on the skin and mucous membranes, not to mention its role in maintaining overall health. Aim for at least eight glasses a day, and remember that caffeine and alcohol can dehydrate you further.

Protein deserves a mention too. It's vital for maintaining muscle mass, which naturally declines with age. A diet rich in high-quality protein from both animal and plant sources can support your physical strength and metabolic health during menopause.

B vitamins, particularly B12 and folate, are critical for energy production and the maintenance of normal brain function. As metabolism and nutrient absorption can change with menopause, ensuring these vitamins are ample in your diet can help maintain your vitality and cognitive function.

Iron is another nutrient to watch. While menopause ends menstruation and the monthly iron loss, maintaining iron-rich diets is beneficial, especially for energy levels and overall vitality. Lean meats, beans, and fortified cereals can all be good sources.

Adapting your diet to meet these nutritional needs doesn't require a radical overhaul but rather conscious choices and small, sustainable changes. The beauty of focusing on these nutrients is not just in their direct benefits but also in the wide array of foods that contain them, allowing for a rich and varied diet.

Empower yourself by taking control of your diet. Consider your plate a palette with which to paint a more vibrant period of life.

Menopause is an opportunity to redefine and rediscover yourself, not just through emotional and spiritual growth, but also by nurturing your body with the essential nutrients it craves.

In the end, embracing menopause with grace and strength does not solely rest on our ability to manage symptoms but in our capacity to thrive during this phase. A diet rich in essential nutrients lays the foundation for health, vitality, and the joy of living fully through menopause and beyond.

Remember, you're not navigating these waters alone. The vast oceans of dietary choices can be overwhelming, but with the right knowledge and a spirit of exploration, you can turn the tide of menopause into a journey of discovery. Let your diet be your ally, a trusted companion on this journey to wellness and empowerment.

Creating a Balanced Diet

Navigating through menopause is akin to embarking on a journey across uncharted waters. Just as a ship requires a balanced load to sail smoothly, our bodies need a balanced diet to transition through menopause with grace. The goal of crafting a balanced diet is not just about managing menopausal symptoms, but about embracing this transformative phase as an opportunity for positive change.

At the heart of a balanced diet is variety. Incorporating a wide range of fruits, vegetables, whole grains, lean proteins, and healthy fats ensures that your body receives a symphony of nutrients. Each nutrient plays a unique role—some may help in managing hot flushes, while others support bone health, mood, and cardiovascular wellness.

Calcium and Vitamin D are pivotal during this stage. As estrogen levels decline, bone density can decrease, heightening the risk of osteoporosis. Dairy products, leafy greens, and fortified foods can be excellent sources of calcium, while Vitamin D can be absorbed through sunlight exposure and fatty fish consumption. It's a dance of getting the right amounts—balance is key.

Magnesium deserves a spotlight for its role in supporting sleep and mood. Nuts, seeds, and whole grains are magnificent sources. Integrating these into your daily meals can help in calming the mind and promoting restful sleep, a precious commodity during menopause.

Omega-3 fatty acids, found in fatty fish, flaxseeds, and walnuts, are known for their anti-inflammatory properties. They're not only beneficial for heart health but may also ease menopausal symptoms such as dry skin and mood swings. Think of them as your dietary allies, bringing a sense of balance and well-being.

Water is the elixir of life, and its importance cannot be overstated, especially now. Keeping hydrated aids in managing hot flushes and supports overall health. Infusing water with fruits or herbs can make it more appealing, ensuring that you drink enough throughout the day.

While it might be tempting to reach for comfort food during times of upheaval, refined sugars and processed foods can exacerbate menopausal symptoms. They can lead to energy crashes and mood swings, obstacles you don't need on this journey. Opting for whole foods over processed options can help stabilise your energy levels and mood.

Portion control is another aspect of creating a balanced diet. Listening to your body's hunger and fullness cues can prevent overeating and help in managing weight, a common concern during menopause. Savour each bite and be mindful of the signals your body sends you.

Experimenting with herbs and spices can make meals more enjoyable without adding unnecessary calories. Many herbs, such as turmeric and ginger, have anti-inflammatory properties, while others, like sage, have been traditionally used to alleviate menopausal symptoms.

Regularly monitoring your diet and adjusting it based on how your body responds is crucial. What works for one person may not work for another. Keeping a food diary can be a helpful tool in identifying foods that trigger symptoms or those that help ease them.

Seeking the guidance of a nutritionist who understands the nuances of menopause can provide personalized dietary advice. This tailored approach can address individual symptoms and dietary preferences, ensuring your diet supports your health and well-being in the most effective way possible.

It's also essential to approach dietary changes with patience and kindness towards yourself. Lifestyle transitions don't happen overnight, and it's okay to have days when you deviate from your planned diet. What matters is persistently striving for balance and moderation.

Lastly, sharing meals with friends and family can not only make eating a more enjoyable experience but also offer support through shared experiences. There's comfort in community, and discussing dietary strategies with others who are navigating similar changes can be incredibly affirming and motivating.

Creating a balanced diet during menopause is much more than just eating the right foods; it's about nurturing your body, respecting its changes, and supporting its journey through this significant life stage. With each mindful choice, you're not just nourishing your body; you're affirming your strength, resilience, and capacity for renewal.

Embrace this transformative period with grace. Let your diet be the foundation upon which you build a healthier, more vibrant version of yourself, ready to welcome the new chapters of your life with open arms and a strengthened spirit.

Chapter 8:
Exercise and Menopause

Embarking on this chapter, it's vital to delve into the transformative power of exercise during menopause. It's not just about maintaining fitness; it's a pivotal strategy for enhancing your overall wellbeing and navigating the menopausal transition with vigour. Exercise isn't a one-size-fits-all remedy; it's about discovering what resonates with your body and lifestyle. The beauty of physical activity lies in its diversity - whether it's a tranquil session of yoga focusing on breath and balance, a brisk walk in nature that clears the mind and uplifts the soul, or more vigorous activities that invigorate the body and sharpen the mind. Each form of movement holds the potential to significantly ease the common symptoms of menopause, from hot flushes to mood swings, bolstering not only physical health but also emotional resilience. Integrating regular exercise into your daily regime can transform it into a potent, empowering tool, aiding in the rebalancing of hormones and fostering a profound connection with your evolving body. This chapter aims to guide you through tailoring your exercise regime, harmoniously blending it with your menopausal journey to foster strength, flexibility, and inner peace. By embracing the role of physical activity, you chart a course through menopause that's not just about enduring change, but thriving through it, emerging with a renewed sense of vitality and joy.

The Role of Physical Activity

Moving into the new chapter of menopause doesn't mean slowing down. In fact, quite the opposite. Exercise during this period isn't just beneficial; it's a potent tool in transforming your menopause journey into a more positive experience. Let's delve deep into how physical activity plays a pivotal role in your life during menopause.

Firstly, exercise serves as a formidable ally against some of the more challenging symptoms of menopause. Hot flushes, night sweats, and mood swings can be mitigated through regular physical activity. It's not merely about the physical act, but about the hormone-like effects exercise induces, helping to naturally balance fluctuating hormone levels.

Moreover, weight management becomes a considerable challenge for many during this stage. As metabolism takes a bit of a nosedive, packing on the pounds becomes easier than shedding them. Here, exercise swoops in as a saviour, boosting your metabolic rate and aiding in weight management. It's about giving your body the best chance to recalibrate and thrive.

It's crucial, however, to acknowledge the diversity in how women experience menopause. For some, vigorous activities can do wonders, while others flourish through gentler, more soothing forms of exercise such as yoga or pilates. The beauty lies in finding what resonates with your body and spirit, thereby crafting a regimen that's uniquely yours.

Let's not forget the sleeping giant – mental health. The capacity of physical activity to enhance mood and mental well-being during menopause cannot be overstated. Exercise releases endorphins, often described as nature's mood lifters, helping combat anxiety and depression. This biochemical shift plays a significant role in navigating the emotional ebbs and flows of menopause.

Bone health is another critical concern post-menopause, with a significant risk increase for osteoporosis. Regular weight-bearing and resistance exercises can fortify bone strength, ensuring that your skeleton remains as resilient as your spirit. The path to prevention, in many cases, is as simple as lacing up your trainers.

Cardiovascular health also demands attention during this phase. Menopause can increase heart disease risk, making exercise not just beneficial but essential. Engaging in activities that get your heart rate up improves cardiovascular fitness and blood pressure, protecting your heart like a precious guard.

Physical activity also has the profound ability to enhance self-esteem and body image, which can take a hit during menopause. Every step, stretch, and lift is a reminder of your strength, resilience, and beauty - mirrored not just in the mirror but more importantly, in your own perception of yourself.

It's important to note that starting an exercise routine, especially if you're new to it, requires a nod from your healthcare provider. Equipped with their guidance, you can embark on this journey safely, ensuring that your endeavours are not just effective but also enjoyable.

Integration of exercise into daily life doesn't demand monumental changes. It starts with small, consistent steps – a brisk walk, a bike ride, or a dance class. The key lies in consistency and gradually increasing intensity and duration as your body adapts.

Setting realistic goals and tracking your progress can hugely impact motivation and commitment. Celebrate every victory, no matter how small. These milestones are the stepping stones to building a healthier, more vibrant you.

Group activities can offer a dual benefit – the support of a community and the motivation to stay on track. Surrounding yourself with like-minded individuals can be incredibly empowering, turning exercise from a solitary endeavour into a shared journey.

Technology, too, has a role to play. Utilise apps and online platforms for guided workouts, tracking capabilities, and virtual support communities. The digital world offers a plethora of resources right at your fingertips, making it easier to integrate physical activity into your busy life.

Remember, transitioning into menopause is a natural, inevitable journey. Yet, how you traverse this path is within your control. Exercise isn't just about physical health; it's a catalyst for a more joyful, empowered, and balanced life during menopause and beyond.

Finally, embrace this time as an opportunity for growth and self-reflection. Menopause, with all its challenges, also opens the door to new beginnings. Embarking on a regimen of physical activity isn't about fighting against the changes in your body but moving in harmony with them. It's about saying yes to yourself, to your health, and to a life lived fully and vibrantly.

So, here's to you – to your strength, your health, and your incredible journey ahead. Let exercise be the companion that walks with you through menopause, offering not just a wealth of health benefits but a source of joy, empowerment, and renewal.

Tailoring Your Exercise Regime

As we embrace this transformative journey through menopause, understanding the pivotal role of exercise isn't just beneficial; it's essential for our overall well-being. It's not merely about staying fit or managing weight, but about crafting a regime that supports our physical and emotional health during this phase. Tailoring your exercise regime to your body's changing needs can significantly enhance your menopause experience.

First and foremost, it's vital to grasp that our bodies respond differently to exercise as we navigate through menopause. The workouts that once felt invigorating might now seem more challenging. This shift isn't a setback but an opportunity to listen to our bodies and adapt our exercise routines accordingly.

Integrating a mix of cardiovascular, strength training, and flexibility exercises can serve as a formidable trio against menopause symptoms. Cardiovascular activities, such as brisk walking or cycling, aren't just excellent for heart health; they also play a crucial role in managing weight and boosting mood. Aiming for at least 150 minutes of moderate-intensity aerobic activity a week can make a noticeable difference.

Strength training, twice a week, is equally crucial. It helps counteract the loss of muscle mass and bone density that can accompany menopause, ultimately reducing the risk of osteoporosis. Moreover, building muscle aids in metabolism regulation, assisting with weight management — a common concern for many post-menopausal women.

Flexibility exercises, including yoga and Pilates, are incredibly beneficial. They not only enhance flexibility and balance but also reduce stress and improve mental well-being. The soothing breathwork and mindful movements can be particularly calming during periods of emotional turbulence.

Listening to your body is key. Some days, you might feel energetic and capable of more intense workouts. On other days, your body might crave gentler, more restorative activities. Honouring these signals is crucial for maintaining a sustainable exercise regime that nurtures rather than depletes your energy.

Hydration and nutrition also play integral roles in tailoring your exercise regime. Staying hydrated is crucial, especially as exercise intensity increases. Additionally, ensuring your diet is rich in essential nutrients supports your physical exertions, helping to maximise the benefits of your workout routine.

Setting realistic goals and expectations is essential. Menopause is a period of change, and as such, our bodies might not always perform as anticipated. Be gentle with yourself and set achievable, flexible goals that encourage a sense of accomplishment without overstraining your body.

Group exercises or classes can offer social and moral support, making exercise an enjoyable and engaging part of your routine. Whether it's joining a walking group or participating in dance classes, being part of a community can significantly enhance motivation and commitment.

Seeking professional advice can be invaluable, especially when constructing a tailored exercise regime for the first time. A fitness coach or physiotherapist who understands the nuances of menopause can provide personalised advice, ensuring your exercise plan is both effective and safe.

Remember, it's not just about physical health. Exercise can profoundly impact your emotional well-being during menopause. Regular physical activity has been shown to alleviate symptoms of depression, anxiety, and stress. It's a powerful tool for enhancing your mood and promoting a positive mental state.

Variety is the spice of life, and this holds true for your exercise routine as well. Mixing up your workouts can prevent boredom and keep you engaged. Experiment with different activities until you find what suits you best, keeping in mind that your preferences may evolve along your menopause journey.

Lastly, celebrate your milestones, no matter how small they might seem. Acknowledging your progress, whether it's increased stamina, strength, or simply consistency in your exercise regime, is vital. It fosters a sense of achievement and motivates continued effort.

In conclusion, tailoring your exercise regime through menopause is a powerful act of self-care. It's an investment in your physical, emotional, and mental health, helping you navigate this transition with strength, resilience, and grace. Embrace this chance to connect with your body in new ways, exploring and adjusting your activities to suit your evolving needs. Let exercise be a source of empowerment, vitality, and joy during your menopause journey.

Chapter 9:
Alternative Therapies and Supplements

In the heart of this transformational journey, many women seek out natural remedies and dietary supplements, hoping to find solace and relief in the gentle arms of Mother Nature. This chapter delves into the world of alternative therapies and supplements, aiming to equip you with the knowledge you need to make informed choices about your menopausal health. It's no secret that the path to finding what works best for your body can be as unique as you are, and here, we explore the plethora of herbal remedies that have been whispered about in holistic circles and scrutinized in scientific studies. From the enigmatic allure of black cohosh to the soothing embrace of evening primrose oil, we'll unpack the evidence behind each remedy's efficacy and safety.

Yet, venturing into the world of supplements requires a vigilant eye. With an overwhelming array of options, discerning which bottles hold promise and which are merely dressed in attractive but empty claims is crucial. We'll guide you through understanding supplement labels, dosages, and the importance of seeking quality products. Moreover, this chapter doesn't shy away from discussing how certain supplements may interact with prescribed medications, a factor often overlooked in the quest for relief. Armed with this knowledge, you're not just a passive spectator but an empowered participant in managing your menopausal symptoms.

While we resonate with the allure of finding a 'natural cure,' it's vital to approach alternative therapies with a balanced perspective. Embracing these remedies doesn't mean turning your back on conventional medicine; rather, it's about harmonizing the two worlds to craft a menopausal journey that's uniquely yours. Let's journey together through the fragrant fields of herbal remedies and the robust shelves of supplements, where science meets tradition, and discover how they can complement your menopausal journey with wisdom, safety, and grace.

Exploring Herbal Remedies

As we journey through the chapters of menopause, exploring herbal remedies becomes a beacon of hope for many. The world of plants offers an extraordinary array of natural solutions that have been nurturing health and wellbeing long before the advent of modern medicine. For women transitioning through menopause, integrating herbal remedies can be a powerful way to alleviate symptoms and enhance vitality.

Understanding the nuances of how each herb interacts with our bodies is crucial. Sage, for instance, stands out as a remarkable herb for its ability to reduce hot flushes and night sweats, two of the most common and challenging symptoms of menopause. Its natural properties help to cool the body and bring a sense of calm to those who consume it.

Another revered plant, Black Cohosh, has been studied for its effectiveness in balancing hormones and providing relief from menopausal symptoms such as mood swings and sleep disturbances. This herb acts as a beacon of light, guiding women through the shadows cast by menopause.

St. John's Wort, praised for its mood-stabilising benefits, becomes a companion for many women facing the emotional waves that menopause can bring. Its ability to gently lift the spirits whilst calming the nerves makes it a valuable ally in maintaining mental well-being during this transitional phase.

The adaptogenic qualities of Ashwagandha cannot be overlooked. This powerful herb supports the body's resilience to stress, a common trigger for menopausal symptoms. By fostering a sense of balance and enhancing energy levels, Ashwagandha empowers women to navigate menopause with grace and strength.

It is, however, imperative to approach herbal remedies with mindfulness and knowledge. Consulting with a healthcare professional before incorporating any new herb into your regimen ensures that these natural remedies work in harmony with your body's unique needs.

Understanding the source of your herbs is equally important. Opting for organically grown and ethically sourced herbs contributes not only to your health but also to the sustenance of our planet. Quality matters, as it directly impacts the potency and effectiveness of these natural remedies.

The preparation of herbal remedies is an art form in itself. Whether you're brewing a cup of soothing tea or incorporating powdered herbs into your meals, the ritual of preparing these remedies can be a meditative and enriching practice, deepening your connection to the healing powers of nature.

Menopause is a journey of transformation. Like any significant life transition, it presents both challenges and opportunities for growth. Herbal remedies offer a path to navigate this change with natural support, aligning with the rhythms of nature to find balance and wellness.

Empowerment comes from making informed choices about your health. By exploring the world of herbal remedies, you're opening the door to a realm of natural resources that can support your menopause journey in profound ways. It's about taking control of your wellbeing, listening to your body, and honouring its transition with care and respect.

The synergy between lifestyle choices and herbal remedies cannot be overstated. Integrating stress-reduction techniques, nourishing foods, and regular physical activity enhances the effectiveness of these natural remedies. Together, they form a comprehensive approach to managing menopause symptoms, embodying the principle of holistic health.

The stories of women who have walked this path before us serve as a source of inspiration and wisdom. Sharing experiences and insights about the healing power of herbs creates a rich tapestry of knowledge, empowering us all to approach menopause with confidence and optimism.

As we delve deeper into the world of herbal remedies, it becomes clear that this path is not just about managing symptoms. It's about embracing menopause as a natural phase of life, one that brings its own gifts and opportunities for growth. With herbs as our allies, we can step into this new chapter with vitality and joy.

The journey through menopause is as unique as each woman who embarks on it. Herbal remedies offer a personalised approach to wellness, allowing each woman to tailor her support according to her specific needs and experiences. In this way, we're not just exploring herbs; we're discovering a deeper connection to ourselves and to the natural world.

In the tapestry of menopause management, herbal remedies emerge as threads of natural wisdom, interwoven with the principles of self-care, empowerment, and ecological responsibility. By exploring these natural offerings, we honour the journey of menopause, embracing it not as an ending but as a vibrant new beginning.

The Science and Safety of Supplements

Navigating the world of supplements during menopause can feel like traversing a landscape filled with promises of relief and well-being. However, understanding the science behind supplements and their safety is crucial. Supplements can offer significant benefits, but they must be approached with the same caution and knowledge as any other health intervention.

The appeal of supplements lies in their potential to fill nutritional gaps, alleviate certain symptoms of menopause, and enhance overall health. Yet, it's essential to recognise that supplements, while beneficial, are not a cure-all. The backbone of health during menopause should be a balanced diet, regular exercise, and adequate sleep. Supplements can, however, play a supportive role in this holistic approach to well-being.

One cannot overemphasize the importance of evidence-based choices. The supplement industry is vast and varied, with products that range from thoroughly researched to anecdotal at best. Women should seek out supplements with a strong backing of scientific research, ideally supported by clinical trials specific to menopausal symptoms. The effectiveness of certain supplements, such as isoflavones for hot flashes or magnesium for sleep, is well-documented, offering a beacon of light for those navigating these common challenges.

However, safety is paramount. The regulation of supplements varies significantly from that of pharmaceuticals. In many regions, supplements are not required to prove efficacy or safety before hitting the market. Consequently, it's imperative to purchase supplements from reputable sources. Look for products that have been independently tested and verified for purity and potency.

Dosage and interactions are also critical considerations. Just because a substance is natural doesn't mean it's harmless in any quantity. Certain supplements can interact with prescription medications, potentially diluting or exacerbating their effects. It's always advisable to consult with a healthcare provider before starting any new supplement, especially for women already taking medications for menopause or other conditions.

In addition to interactions, the timing and duration of supplement use should be carefully considered. Some supplements are intended for short-term relief of symptoms, while others may be geared towards long-term health benefits. Understanding the recommended duration of use and monitoring the body's response over time is crucial.

It's also worth noting the role of individual biology in supplement efficacy. What works miracles for one woman might have little to no effect on another. Genetic factors, lifestyle, and the specific symptoms experienced during menopause all play a role in how supplements impact an individual. Starting with low doses and gradually increasing, if necessary, can help gauge personal tolerance and effectiveness.

Sensitivity to certain ingredients is another concern. Fillers, binders, and coloring agents in supplements can sometimes cause adverse reactions. Reading labels carefully and choosing products with minimal additives can help minimize these risks.

While exploring supplements, the importance of a nutrient-rich diet cannot be understated. Supplements are meant to supplement, not replace, the nutrients obtained from food. A diet rich in fruits, vegetables, whole grains, and lean proteins provides a solid foundation upon which supplements can build.

The evolving landscape of menopause research continually brings new insights into effective supplements. Staying informed through trustworthy sources and healthcare professionals ensures that one's supplement regimen remains up to date and conducive to health and well-being.

Mindfulness and patience are key. The effects of supplements can be subtle and gradual. It's important to listen to the body and give it time to adjust. Tracking symptoms before and after starting supplements can provide valuable feedback on their effectiveness and help refine one's approach.

Focusing on quality over quantity is essential. Rather than overwhelming the body with a plethora of supplements, prioritizing a few based on individual needs and evidence of their benefits can be more effective. This approach not only simplifies one's regimen but also minimizes the risk of adverse interactions and side effects.

Exploring the world of supplements can be an empowering part of the menopause journey. With an informed and cautious approach, supplements can effectively complement traditional therapies and lifestyle changes, helping women navigate this transformative phase with grace and strength.

In conclusion, while the promise of supplements is compelling, their incorporation into a menopausal health strategy must be done thoughtfully. Armed with knowledge, guided by evidence, and supported by professional advice, women can safely explore supplements as a valuable ally in their quest for wellness during menopause and beyond.

Chapter 10:
Medical Treatments and Considerations

As we journey deeper into the landscape of menopause, it's paramount that we explore the avenues of medical treatments and considerations with open minds and hearts. The transition through menopause is as unique as the individual experiencing it, thus the approach to managing symptoms and enhancing well-being must be equally personalised. Delving into **Hormone Replacement Therapy (HRT)**, we weigh its pros and cons, understanding that while it offers relief for many, it's not a one-size-fits-all solution. Equally, the exploration of **non-hormonal medical options** reveals a spectrum of alternatives that can mitigate symptoms while aligning with your body's needs and preferences. Through this chapter, we embark on a journey to demystify these treatments, aiming to equip you with the knowledge to make informed decisions. Informed by the latest research and expert insights, we navigate this terrain, emphasising that empowerment in menopause isn't just about the challenges we overcome, but also about the choices we make to ensure our journey is marked by strength, grace, and informed consent. Let's embrace this chapter of our lives, not as a time of loss, but as an opportunity for profound growth and well-being, supported by the best medical care tailored to our individual journeys.

Hormone Replacement Therapy (HRT): Pros and Cons

Hormone Replacement Therapy (HRT) stands as one of the most discussed topics when it comes to managing menopause. For many women, HRT offers a beacon of hope, possibly turning the tide against some of the more challenging symptoms associated with this natural stage of life. Understanding the pros and cons of this treatment is crucial in making an informed decision that aligns with one's health aspirations and concerns.

At its core, HRT seeks to replenish the body with estrogen and, in some cases, progesterone, which taper off during menopause. This decline in hormones is what brings about many of the symptoms that can, at times, deeply affect a woman's quality of life. From hot flushes to mood swings and decreased libido, the impacts are wide-ranging. By addressing the hormonal imbalance, HRT can offer significant relief, enhancing daily function and overall wellbeing.

One of the most persuasive arguments for HRT is its effectiveness against hot flushes, which are among the most common and debilitating symptoms of menopause. Numerous studies have shown that HRT can dramatically reduce both the frequency and intensity of hot flushes, providing a much-needed respite for countless women.

Beyond managing hot flushes, HRT has also been shown to be effective in improving sleep quality. Menopause can turn a good night's sleep into a fleeting wish for many, with sleep disturbances being a common complaint. By stabilising hormone levels, HRT can help in promoting a more restful sleep, making it easier to recharge and tackle the day ahead.

Moreover, HRT's benefits extend into the realms of mood stabilisation and mental health. The fluctuating hormone levels during menopause can take a toll on emotional wellbeing, leading to mood swings and even depression in some cases. HRT has been linked to improved mood and cognitive function, making it a vital consideration for those struggling in this area.

However, the journey through menopause is deeply personal, and what works for one woman may not for another. It's also essential to delve into the cons of HRT, understanding that its use comes with considerations that must be carefully weighed. One of the most significant concerns revolves around the potential increased risk of certain health conditions, including breast cancer, stroke, and blood clots.

The relationship between HRT and breast cancer risk, in particular, has been the subject of intense research and debate. While some studies suggest a slight increase in risk, especially with long-term use, the picture is complex and influenced by factors such as the type of HRT, the dosage, and the individual's health history. It's a topic that necessitates a nuanced discussion with a healthcare provider, taking into account personal risk factors and family history.

Considering cardiovascular health, the consensus has shifted over the years. Initially, concerns were raised about a possible link between HRT and increased risks of heart disease and stroke. However, more recent studies suggest that the timing of HRT initiation might be key, with early use (typically within ten years of menopause onset) potentially offering some protective benefits against heart disease.

The risk of blood clots is another factor that cannot be ignored. HRT, particularly in its oral form, has been associated with a higher risk of developing venous thromboembolism (VTE), including deep vein thrombosis (DVT) and pulmonary embolism (PE). As with other risks, this necessitates a tailored approach to HRT, considering alternative methods of administration such as patches or gels, which have been shown to have a lower risk of VTE.

Another dimension to consider is the impact of HRT on bone health. Osteoporosis becomes a more pressing concern as women age, and the drop in estrogen levels during menopause can accelerate bone density loss. HRT has been shown to reduce the risk of osteoporosis and related fractures, underscoring its potential benefit in protecting skeletal health as women transition through menopause and beyond.

Understanding the full spectrum of HRT's pros and cons requires an open dialogue with healthcare professionals who can provide personalised advice based on individual health profiles and concerns. It's also about listening to one's body and weighing how the benefits stack up against the potential risks.

In navigating the decision-making process, it's imperative to consider not just the physical dimensions of menopause and HRT but also the emotional and psychological aspects. For many women, the choice to use HRT is not solely about alleviating physical symptoms but about seeking a pathway to reclaim control over their bodies and lives during a time of profound change.

Importantly, the narrative around HRT and menopause is shifting. We are moving towards a model of care that respects the agency of women, prioritizing informed choice and tailored approaches over one-size-fits-all solutions. This evolution in perspective is a welcome change, empowering women to make decisions that align with their health goals, values, and visions for their future.

In conclusion, HRT offers a powerful tool in the management of menopause, with the potential to significantly improve quality of life. However, its use is not without complexities and requires a careful consideration of its pros and cons. As we stand at this crossroads, let us embrace the knowledge we have, engage in open conversations with healthcare professionals, and make choices that bring us closer to the life we envision for ourselves as we navigate this natural, albeit challenging, phase of life.

Non-Hormonal Medical Options

Transitioning through menopause can be like navigating through a maze, with each turn presenting its unique challenges. While Hormone Replacement Therapy (HRT) is a well-known path for many, it's not the only route on the map. For women seeking alternative avenues, the realm of non-hormonal medical options offers promising paths worth exploring.

At the heart of non-hormonal treatments is the understanding that menopause, while a natural phase, brings with it symptoms that can significantly impact one's quality of life. From hot flushes to mood swings, the physical and emotional upheavals require attention and care. As we delve into these options, it's crucial to remember that each woman's journey is distinct, and what works for one may not for another.

One of the first ports of call for managing hot flushes and night sweats without hormones is the use of certain antidepressants. Medications such as SSRIs and SNRIs, originally designed to treat depression, have been found to alleviate these symptoms in some women. It's a fascinating example of how medications can have beneficial 'side effects', providing relief in unexpected ways.

Beyond mood management, non-hormonal options also extend to addressing the atrophy and dryness of the vaginal tissues, which can lead to discomfort during sexual activity. Vaginal moisturizers and lubricants can provide significant relief. These products, readily available, can enhance comfort and intimacy, helping to maintain the quality of one's sexual health and relationships during menopause.

Further, for those experiencing more severe genitourinary symptoms, prescription treatments such as ospemifene offer a hormone-free option. Designed to specifically target the tissues of the vagina, it can improve symptoms of atrophy without the use of traditional hormone therapy.

The landscape of non-hormonal treatments also includes options for bone health, a major concern for many women post-menopause. Medications such as bisphosphonates help in maintaining bone density and preventing osteoporosis, offering a preventive approach to long-term skeletal health.

For women grappling with the increased cardiovascular risks post-menopause, a combination of lifestyle modifications and medications can help manage blood pressure and cholesterol levels. Here, the focus shifts to a holistic approach, blending medication with dietary changes and physical activity to protect heart health.

In addressing mood swings and mental well-being, Cognitive Behavioural Therapy (CBT) emerges as a powerful tool. Without the reliance on medications, CBT offers strategies to manage anxiety and depression, teaching coping mechanisms that can greatly improve the menopausal experience.

Moreover, the journey through menopause is also an opportunity to explore the impact of complementary therapies. While not 'medical' in the traditional sense, practices such as acupuncture and mindfulness can offer significant relief for symptoms like hot flushes, proving that relief comes in many forms.

It's vital to approach menopause with a spirit of exploration and openness, willing to try different strategies to find what truly works for you. Engage in conversations with healthcare providers about these non-hormonal options, armed with the knowledge that you are not limited to a single path but have many avenues to explore.

Remember, navigating menopause is not just about managing symptoms but about embracing a transformative phase of life. Each treatment chosen is a step towards not just symptom relief but also self-discovery, resilience, and empowerment.

While the journey may seem daunting at times, the array of non-hormonal options offers a beacon of hope. They serve as a reminder that menopause, with all its complexities, also brings an opportunity to prioritize oneself, making health-conscious decisions that resonate with one's body and lifestyle.

As you consider these options, let the guiding principle be one of self-care and informed choice. Menopause is not an end but a transition, an evolution into a period of life that can be as fulfilling and vibrant as any other. With the right support and treatments, it's possible to navigate this journey with grace and strength, embracing the transformation with an open heart and a spirit of positivity.

In conclusion, the voyage through menopause, while unique for every woman, need not be travelled alone or without aid. The panorama of non-hormonal medical options offers a testament to the advances in healthcare, ensuring that every woman has access to the support and treatments necessary to transition through this phase with confidence and well-being. Embrace this journey as an opportunity for growth and self-care, knowing that a multitude of paths lie before you, each promising relief, renewal, and resilience.

Chapter 11:
The Heart of the Matter: Cardiovascular Health

As we turn the page to a pivotal chapter in our journey, "The Heart of the Matter: Cardiovascular Health" beckons us to focus our attentions inward, to the very core of our being—the heart. It's a stark reality that women facing menopause are met with an increased risk for cardiovascular diseases, a fact that underscores the importance of understanding the intricacies of heart health during this phase. Yet, here lies an opportunity wrapped in a challenge; to not only comprehend the risks but to actively engage in prevention and management strategies that can profoundly impact our wellbeing. It's empowering to learn that through informed dietary choices, dedicated physical activity, and stress management, we can wield considerable influence over our cardiovascular health. This chapter isn't just about recognizing the increased risks; it's a call to action, a guide designed to arm you with the knowledge and tools necessary to navigate this terrain with confidence. The path to maintaining a healthy heart amidst menopause is multifaceted, involving a balanced synergy between medical guidance and lifestyle adjustments. I invite you to journey with me as we uncover the secrets to safeguarding your heart's health, ensuring that it continues to beat with strength and vitality, empowering you to embrace every moment of this transformative phase with grace and vigour.

Understanding Risks

As we embark on the journey towards understanding the risks associated with cardiovascular health during menopause, it's essential to recognise the shifts that occur within our bodies. Just as menopause signals a transformative phase in a woman's life, so too does it alter the landscape of her cardiovascular risk profile. It's a time of profound change, where being informed can empower us to take proactive steps towards safeguarding our heart health.

The decline in estrogen levels associated with menopause has been linked to an increased risk of cardiovascular disease. This hormone once played a protective role in maintaining the elasticity of blood vessels, facilitating smooth blood flow. As levels drop, women may face a higher risk of developing conditions such as hypertension or atherosclerosis, known precursors to more serious cardiovascular health issues.

Moreover, menopause brings with it changes in body composition, often leading to increased visceral fat. This type of fat is particularly concerning as it's not only associated with an elevated risk of heart disease but also with diabetes and stroke. Recognising these changes is the first step towards mitigating their impact on our heart health.

It's also important to be mindful of the silent nature of cardiovascular disease. Many women may not experience overt symptoms until a significant health event occurs. This underscores the importance of regular health screenings and paying attention to even subtle changes in our bodies and energy levels. Being proactive can quite literally save lives.

Another key factor to consider is the role of lifestyle choices on cardiovascular health during menopause. Diet, exercise, and stress management are not just general wellness recommendations; they are cardiovascular health imperatives. A balanced diet rich in nutrients supports heart health, while regular physical activity improves cardiovascular fitness and weight management aids in reducing the risk associated with increased visceral fat.

Stress, too, plays a significant role in cardiovascular risk. The emotional and psychological changes that accompany menopause can heighten stress levels, which in turn can impact heart health. Finding effective stress management techniques, therefore, isn't just beneficial for our mental well-being; it's critical for our physical health as well.

Let's not overlook the impact of smoking and excessive alcohol consumption. Both have been shown to exacerbate the risk of cardiovascular diseases. If there was ever a time to quit or reduce these habits, menopause is it. Making these changes might be challenging, but the benefits to heart health are undeniable.

Family history is another crucial aspect of understanding cardiovascular risks. A family history of heart disease can increase your risk, making it even more important to focus on controllable lifestyle factors and to communicate openly with your healthcare provider about your heart health.

However, it's not all doom and gloom. Menopause represents a powerful opportunity for renewal and change. Educating ourselves about these risks equips us to make informed decisions that can have a profound impact on our cardiovascular health. The choices we make today regarding our lifestyle, diet, and activity levels can dramatically influence our heart health tomorrow.

It's also worth noting the importance of a supportive healthcare team. A partnership with knowledgeable healthcare providers who understand the nuances of menopause and cardiovascular health can make a significant difference. They can offer tailored advice, recommend regular screenings and tests, and help you navigate the complexities of managing risk factors.

Prevention is undeniably better than cure. Adopting a heart-healthy lifestyle before significant symptoms or issues arise can set the stage for a healthier post-menopausal life. Simple adjustments to diet, incorporating regular physical activity, and maintaining a healthy weight can be potent preventative measures.

Let's also talk about the power of education and community. Sharing knowledge and experiences with other women going through similar changes can be incredibly empowering. It fosters a sense of community and support that is invaluable during this phase of life. Women should be encouraged to speak openly about their health concerns, including cardiovascular health, and seek support.

In summary, understanding the cardiovascular risks associated with menopause is crucial for every woman. It's a call to action, urging us to pay closer attention to our bodies, make healthier lifestyle choices, and seek support when needed. Remember, you're not alone in this journey. Together, we can navigate these changes with knowledge, strength, and grace, ensuring that our hearts remain as strong and vibrant as our spirits.

So, let's embrace this period of transformation with open hearts and minds. Let's make informed decisions that prioritise our cardiovascular health, understanding that in doing so, we're not just looking after our physical well-being, but we're also nurturing our overall quality of life. Menopause is not an end but a new beginning – a chance to reinvent ourselves with health, wisdom, and empowerment at the forefront.

In a way, taking charge of our cardiovascular health during menopause symbolises taking charge of our lives. It's an act of self-care, self-respect, and, ultimately, self-love. And in this journey towards a healthier heart, remember: every step taken is a victory, every informed choice a triumph. Here's to our hearts, may they beat strongly and healthily as we navigate this transformative chapter of our lives together.

Prevention and Management Strategies

Navigating the transformative stage of menopause with grace and strength involves understanding the heart of the matter - our cardiovascular health. It's well-known that as women transition through menopause, changes in our cardiovascular system present new challenges, but also opportunities for profound empowerment through prevention and management strategies. Let's embark on this journey together, equipped with knowledge and inspired to take action.

Firstly, the cornerstone of cardiovascular health during menopause is a balanced diet. A diet rich in fruits, vegetables, whole grains, and lean protein sources isn't just about weight maintenance; these foods are the allies of your heart. They help manage cholesterol levels, reduce blood pressure, and decrease the risk of heart disease. Integrating omega-3 fatty acids, found in oily fish and flaxseeds, can further protect your heart by reducing inflammation and increasing good cholesterol levels.

Moving your body daily is not just a mantra for fitness enthusiasts but a lifeline for your heart. Exercise, especially aerobic activities like walking, cycling, or swimming, strengthens your heart muscle and improves circulation. It's also a fabulous way to manage stress and improve mood, offering a triple-edged sword for combating heart disease. Tailoring your exercise regime to something you enjoy ensures you'll stick with it long-term. Remember, consistency over intensity.

Stress, often overlooked, plays a significant role in cardiovascular health. Developing stress-reduction techniques such as mindfulness, meditation, or yoga can lower blood pressure and heart rate, easing the burden on your heart. Viewing these practices not as another task on your to-do list but as a refuge can transform your approach to stress management.

Regular health screenings become increasingly important as we age. Monitoring blood pressure, cholesterol levels, and blood sugar can catch potential problems early. Don't view these check-ups as something ominous but as an act of self-respect, keeping you in tune with your body's needs and changes.

Smoking cessation is a non-negotiable. If you smoke, stopping is perhaps the most powerful change you can make for your heart. It's never too late to quit, and the benefits start immediately. Your risk of heart disease significantly drops even within the first year of quitting. Consider seeking support through programs designed to help you stop smoking; there is strength in asking for help.

Limited alcohol consumption also plays a vital role. While moderate alcohol intake might have some heart benefits for certain individuals, excessive drinking can raise blood pressure and harm the heart. Finding a balance and knowing your limits is crucial.

Weight management through a combination of diet and exercise keeps your heart healthy by preventing undue stress on it and reducing the risk of other conditions like diabetes, which is closely linked to heart disease. However, approach weight management with compassion and realism, focusing on gradual changes that feel sustainable rather than drastic overhauls.

Embracing a heart-healthy lifestyle also means finding joy in the journey. Whether it's experimenting with new recipes that are good for your heart, discovering a passion for a new form of exercise, or taking solace in stress-reduction techniques, joy is a powerful motivator. Allow yourself to explore, change, and find new ways to keep your heart healthy.

Understand that hormone replacement therapy (HRT) can play a complex role in cardiovascular health. For some, it may offer benefits; for others, risks. Discussing your personal risk factors and concerns with a healthcare provider ensures you make informed decisions tailored to your unique health profile.

Building a support network of friends, family, and healthcare providers creates a holistic approach to cardiovascular health. Sharing your goals, successes, and challenges not only provides accountability but also ensures you have a cheering squad rooting for every step you take towards a healthier heart.

Supplements and alternative therapies can complement traditional approaches to heart health. However, approach these with a critical eye and in consultation with healthcare professionals. Not all supplements are created equal, and some may interact with medications.

Remember, prevention and management of cardiovascular health is not about fear but about empowerment. It's about making choices that respect and honor this incredible journey through menopause and beyond. It's not just about adding years to your life but adding life to your years.

Embrace this time of transition as an opportunity to reevaluate and renew your commitment to heart health. Let go of old habits that no longer serve you and open your heart to new practices that uplift and nurture your well-being.

In conclusion, the pathway to a healthy heart during and after menopause is multifaceted but deeply rewarding. It's an invitation to care for yourself with love, patience, and determination. Each step you take towards improving your cardiovascular health is a step towards a vibrant, empowered life where menopause is celebrated as a chapter of renewal and strength.

Chapter 12:
Bone Integrity and Menopause

As we journey through the chapters of our lives, menopause stands as a significant milestone, heralding changes that extend beyond the cessation of menstruation. Among these, the impact on bone health is paramount, signalling a time when our vigilance towards maintaining bone integrity must intensify. With the decline in oestrogen levels, our bones may become more susceptible to loss and fracture, an ailment most commonly recognised as osteoporosis. Yet, this chapter in our story need not be one of vulnerability but can be an empowering narrative of prevention and resilience.

Understanding the symbiotic relationship between menopause and bone health prompts us to adopt lifestyle choices that fortify our skeletal framework—choices such as optimising our diet with calcium and vitamin D, engaging in regular weight-bearing and muscle-strengthening exercises, and when appropriate, considering medical treatments that support bone density. It's a testament to the strength within us, the capability to adapt and thrive amidst the tides of change. Amidst these strategic efforts, we also discover the importance of timely bone density screening, a tool that offers us insight into our bone health status, enabling us to act proactively.

Let this chapter serve as a beacon, guiding us towards practices that not only uphold our bone health but reinforce our overall well-being. Embracing this phase with informed choices allows us to stand strong, literally and metaphorically, as we navigate the waters of menopause. It's a period for self-care, a testament to the enduring strength and adaptability of women. With each step forward, let us lean into the journey with confidence, acknowledging that in safeguarding our bone integrity, we cultivate a foundation of health that will support us in the vibrant chapters to come.

Osteoporosis: Risk and Prevention

As women, our journey through menopause is not just a passage of time or a series of hot flushes and mood swings. It's a profound chapter in our lives where our bodies undergo significant transformations, one of which affects our bones. Yes, we're talking about osteoporosis, a condition that might not manifest with obvious symptoms, yet silently impacts many postmenopausal women. But let's not approach this with trepidation; rather, let's empower ourselves with knowledge and strategies for prevention.

Osteoporosis, or the thinning of bone mass and density, often sneaks up unnoticed until a sudden fall results in a fracture. It's a sobering fact that postmenopausal women are at a higher risk due to the decrease in estrogen levels, a hormone critical to bone health. However, this realization isn't a verdict but a call to action. By understanding the risk factors and embracing preventive measures, we can take significant strides towards safeguarding our bone integrity.

Firstly, let's consider the role of calcium and vitamin D, the cornerstone nutrients for bone health. Adequate daily intake of calcium-rich foods and vitamin D - either through diet, supplements, or sun exposure - is crucial. Yet, it's not just about consumption but also about absorption. Factors such as vitamin K2 also play a vital role in ensuring calcium is deposited in our bones and not in our arteries.

Exercise, particularly weight-bearing and resistance training, is another powerful tool in our arsenal against osteoporosis. Engaging in regular physical activity not only strengthens our muscles but also improves bone density. It's a beautiful synergy where our body supports strength building in response to the demands placed on it.

Moreover, lifestyle choices such as smoking cessation and moderating alcohol intake can have a positive impact on bone health. These habits not only affect our overall well-being but specifically our skeletal system's resilience against age-related decline.

In addition to lifestyle adjustments, hormone replacement therapy (HRT) can be a viable option for some women to mitigate the risk of osteoporosis. This treatment, while not suitable for everyone, can help maintain bone density by supplementing estrogen levels, highlighting the individual nature of our menopausal journey and the importance of tailored medical advice.

A pivotal aspect of prevention is early detection. Regular bone density scans, as recommended by healthcare providers, can offer crucial insights into our bone health, enabling interventions at an earlier stage, if necessary.

Also noteworthy is the contribution of certain medications that can either aid in increasing bone mass or slowing bone loss. Again, this underlines the need for a dialogue with healthcare professionals to explore options that align with individual health profiles and risk factors.

Dietary patterns play a significant role in bone health. A diet rich in fruits, vegetables, and lean proteins supports overall health and provides key nutrients like magnesium and phosphorus, essential for bone integrity. This isn't about strict diets but about mindful, balanced eating habits that nourish our bodies from within.

Stress management is another critical factor. Chronic stress can lead to elevated cortisol levels, which have been linked to bone density reduction. Embracing strategies for mental and emotional well-being can, therefore, indirectly contribute to healthier bones.

Hydration is often overlooked when discussing bone health. Adequate water intake is essential for all bodily functions, including the maintenance of healthy joints and the effective absorption of calcium.

Let's not forget about community and support networks. Sharing experiences and strategies with other women going through similar journeys can be incredibly empowering. It reminds us that we're not alone and that collective wisdom can be a source of strength and inspiration.

While genetics do play a role in our predisposition to osteoporosis, it's empowering to realize the significant impact our lifestyle choices have on our health outcomes. We are not utterly at the mercy of our DNA; we have the agency to influence our well-being positively.

Lastly, the journey towards preventing osteoporosis is not a race nor does it boast an overnight fix. It's a commitment to ourselves, to embrace habits that foster strength, resilience, and vitality. It's about making informed choices today that pave the way for a healthier tomorrow.

In summary, menopause presents us with challenges, but it also offers us opportunities to reevaluate, recalibrate, and reinforce our health practices. Osteoporosis prevention is not just about bones; it's an integral part of a holistic approach towards a vibrant and fulfilling postmenopausal life. As we navigate this chapter, let's do so with confidence, supported by the knowledge that our actions can vastly improve our quality of life. So here's to strong bones, enduring spirits, and a menopause journey embraced with grace and strength.

Strength from Within: Lifestyle for Bone Health

As we navigate the journey of menopause together, it's paramount that we turn our focus inward, to the very foundation of our strength - our bones. Menopause, while a natural transition, brings with it changes that can affect our bone density and overall skeletal health. However, with targeted lifestyle choices, we can fortify our bones from within, ensuring we remain strong and resilient.

One of the cornerstones of maintaining bone health during and after menopause is nutrition. It's about much more than just drinking milk or taking a calcium supplement. Our bodies are complex systems that require a variety of nutrients to build and maintain strong bones. Calcium is undeniably important, but it's vitally important to ensure you're also getting sufficient vitamin D, which helps your body absorb calcium, alongside other key nutrients such as magnesium and vitamin K.

Moreover, protein plays a critical role in bone health. Incorporating lean protein sources into your diet, like fish, poultry, and legumes, can offer significant benefits. A balanced diet rich in fruits and vegetables also contributes to the minerals and vitamins necessary for bone density. It's not simply about what we add to our diets, but what we might need to reduce or eliminate, such as excessive sodium and caffeine, which can impede calcium absorption.

Physical activity is another pillar supporting strong bones. Weight-bearing and resistance exercises are particularly effective, as they stimulate bone formation. Activities like walking, dancing, yoga, and lifting weights not only strengthen bones but also improve balance and coordination, reducing the risk of falls and fractures.

Smoking and excessive alcohol consumption can severely impair bone health. These habits can increase bone loss, leading to a higher risk of osteoporosis. Making the choice to reduce or quit smoking and limit alcohol intake can significantly impact your bone density positively.

Understanding your personal risk factors for osteoporosis is also crucial. Family history, body frame size, and certain medical conditions and medications can affect bone health. Discussing these factors with your healthcare provider can help you take proactive steps tailored to your specific needs.

Hydration, often overlooked, is surprisingly significant for bone health. Dehydration can reduce the blood's ability to supply the necessary nutrients to our bones. Ensuring you're drinking sufficient water day-to-day is a simple yet effective way to support your skeletal structure.

Stress management plays an unexpected role in bone health as well. Chronic stress can lead to elevated cortisol levels, which has been associated with bone density loss. Embracing stress-reduction practices such as meditation, deep breathing exercises, or mindful walking can indirectly benefit your bones.

Monitoring bone density through medical check-ups can catch potential issues early. Bone density tests can offer a snapshot of your bone health, enabling you and your doctor to make informed decisions regarding your lifestyle and any need for medication.

Supplements can also play a role in bone health, especially when it's challenging to get enough nutrients from diet alone. Calcium and vitamin D are the most commonly recommended supplements, but it's important to consult with a healthcare provider for personalised advice, ensuring you take the right types and amounts.

Equally, staying informed about the latest research and recommendations on menopause and bone health is pivotal. Medical science evolves, and staying updated enables you to make the best decisions for your health.

Understanding the link between hormonal changes during menopause and bone density is critical. Estrogen, which declines during menopause, plays a key role in maintaining bone density. Hormone Replacement Therapy (HRT) might be beneficial for some women in reducing bone loss. However, it's essential to have an in-depth discussion with your healthcare provider about the risks and benefits specific to your health profile.

Maintaining a healthy weight is beneficial for bone health as well. Extreme weight loss or being underweight can increase the risk of osteoporosis, while excess weight can put unnecessary stress on the bones. Finding a balanced, healthy weight through nutrition and exercise is a key strategy for protecting your bones.

Lastly, embracing a positive mindset towards menopause and aging can significantly influence your lifestyle choices and health outcomes. Viewing this time as a period of growth and renewal encourages proactive steps towards not just maintaining bone health, but improving overall well-being.

Fortifying our bones from within requires a holistic approach, integrating mindful nutrition, adequate exercise, lifestyle adjustments, and informed medical choices. As we embrace these practices, we're not just caring for our bones; we're building a stronger, empowered version of ourselves, ready to thrive through menopause and beyond.

Chapter 13:
Skin and Hair: The Outer Reflection

As we journey through the chapters of our lives, the tale of menopause unfolds with unique narratives for each of us, casting a spotlight on our skin and hair as potent symbols of this transformative era. The metamorphosis experienced by our bodies isn't confined within; it mirrors on our skin and dances through our hair, narrating stories of change, resilience, and beauty reborn. Embracing these shifts requires an understanding that skin might become more prone to dryness, losing some of its youthful elasticity, and hair may whisper tales of thinning or altered textures. Yet, this chapter isn't about mourning changes but about empowering you with strategies and insights to nourish, protect, and celebrate your skin and hair. By weaving targeted nutrition, tailored skincare routines, and gentle, loving acceptance into our daily lives, we can reflect the inner strength and grace we possess. It's about seeing beyond the superficial, recognising these changes as an outer reflection of a profound internal journey and embracing them with care, dignity, and pride. This isn't merely a transition; it's an opportunity to redefine beauty on our own terms, asserting that our skin and hair are not just tales of times past but vibrant declarations of the present and future chapters yet to be written.

Navigating Changes in Skin

As we journey through the chapters of our lives, entering the menopause phase brings about transformations that are both profound and empowering. Among these changes, our skin - the largest organ and the outer reflection of our inner health and vitality - undergoes its own unique set of challenges. It's crucial to understand and embrace these changes, equipping ourselves with knowledge and strategies to navigate this transition gracefully.

The decline in oestrogen levels during menopause directly impacts our skin's appearance, elasticity, and moisture levels. You might notice your skin becomes drier, less plump, and more susceptible to fine lines and wrinkles. This isn't just about vanity; it's about understanding the physiological shifts occurring within and responding with care and compassion.

Hydration is your skin's best friend at this stage. Internally, increasing your water intake is fundamental. Externally, investing in a good-quality, hydrating moisturiser can make a significant difference. Look for products containing hyaluronic acid, which has a remarkable ability to retain moisture, and don't forget to nourish your skin at night when the regeneration process is at its peak.

Moreover, the thinning of the skin makes it more vulnerable to UV damage. Sun protection isn't just for younger years; it's essential throughout life. Opt for a broad-spectrum sunscreen to protect against both UVA and UVB rays, even on cloudy days. Remember, sun damage is cumulative, and safeguarding your skin is a key prevention strategy against premature ageing and skin cancer.

Nutrition plays a pivotal role in skin health. Foods rich in antioxidants, omega-3 fatty acids, and vitamins can fortify your skin against environmental stresses and support cellular repair. Embrace a rainbow diet filled with fruits, vegetables, nuts, and seeds to provide your skin with the nutrients it needs to thrive.

Menopause might also bring about an increase in skin sensitivity and the potential for rosacea or acne to reemerge or worsen. It's vital to reassess your skincare routine and possibly streamline it. Avoid harsh, irritating ingredients and opt for gentle, non-comedogenic products that support skin's natural barrier function.

Exercise, too, plays a surprising role in skin health. Regular physical activity boosts circulation, which in turn encourages the detoxification process and delivers oxygen and nutrients more efficiently to the skin. This can help to promote a healthier, more radiant complexion.

Don't underestimate the power of sleep. It's called 'beauty sleep' for a reason. During deep sleep, the repair and regeneration of skin cells are accelerated. Aim for 7-9 hours of quality sleep per night, establishing a relaxing bedtime routine to aid in drifting off more easily.

The psychological impact of skin changes shouldn't be ignored. Our skin is integral to our self-image and confidence. It's natural to experience a range of emotions as you navigate these changes. Acknowledge these feelings, but also remember to extend kindness and patience to yourself. This chapter in your life is a profound journey of transformation and renewal.

Professional treatments, such as laser therapy, microdermabrasion, or chemical peels, can be beneficial for some women. However, these should be considered carefully and always discussed with a dermatologist who understands the nuances of skin care during menopause.

Supplements can also support skin health. Ingredients like collagen peptides, vitamin E, and selenium have shown promise in improving skin elasticity and texture. Still, it's essential to consult with a healthcare provider before adding any new supplements to your routine.

Remember, skin care is deeply personal. What works for one person may not for another. It's about listening to your skin, understanding its needs, and adapting your approach accordingly. Be open to trying new things but do so with mindfulness and intention.

Community and shared experiences can also be an invaluable resource. Talking with friends or joining a support group can provide insights and tips that have worked for others navigating similar changes. There's comfort in knowing you're not alone in this journey.

Ultimately, these changes in our skin are a natural part of the aging process and, more specifically, the menopause transition. With the right care, knowledge, and attitude, you can navigate this phase with confidence and grace. Your skin, like you, is resilient and capable of incredible renewal. Embracing this chapter with an optimistic and proactive mindset is the key to not just surviving but thriving.

In closing, as you navigate the changes in your skin, remember that this journey is an opportunity for growth and empowerment. Menopause is not an end but a beginning, a chance to redefine your relationship with your body and celebrate its strength, resilience, and beauty. With compassion, care, and a dash of courage, you can emerge through this transition more vibrant and radiant than ever before.

Hair Health and Menopause

The journey through menopause is as much about the changes we can see as about those we feel. Among the most visible transformations, and perhaps one of the most disconcerting for many, is the change in hair health and density. Menopause can herald a time when your hair may not seem as full or vibrant as it once was. However, understanding what's happening and arming yourself with strategies to support hair health can turn concern into confidence.

Firstly, it's essential to recognize that fluctuating hormone levels play a significant role in these changes. Estrogen and progesterone, which support hair growth and maintenance, decrease during menopause. At the same time, androgens, or male hormones, can increase, potentially leading to hair thinning on your head and more hair in places you wouldn't expect or desire.

It can be disheartening to find clumps of hair in the shower or your brush, but it's vital to approach this phase with a mindset of care and positivity rather than distress. You're not alone in this experience, and there are myriad ways to manage and mitigate these changes. Diet, for example, is a cornerstone of hair health. Nutrients like protein, iron, omega-3 fatty acids, and vitamins D and B12 are crucial for maintaining healthy hair. Incorporating a balanced diet rich in these nutrients can help support hair strength and growth.

Scalp care too takes on new importance during menopause. A healthy scalp promotes healthy hair. Gentle, regular massaging of the scalp can stimulate blood flow, while choosing the right shampoo and conditioner for your hair type can keep the scalp clean and hydrated.

Sometimes, what's needed is a fresh approach to hair care. Heat styling, harsh chemicals, and tight hairstyles can all exacerbate hair thinning. Embracing your natural hair texture and exploring gentler styling methods can not only protect your hair but also reinvigorate your relationship with it.

For those seeking further support, a range of treatments and supplements are available. Topical minoxidil, for example, is FDA-approved for female pattern hair loss and can be effective in stimulating regrowth. Meanwhile, biotin and other over-the-counter hair supplements have shown promise in supporting hair health, though it's wise to consult with a healthcare provider before starting any new supplement regimen.

The psychological impact of hair changes should not be underestimated. Society places a great deal of emphasis on hair as a symbol of youth and vitality, which can make the experience of hair thinning particularly challenging. Engaging with a supportive community, whether online or in person, can provide solace and strength. Sharing stories and strategies helps not just in practical terms but in reinforcing the message that you're not navigating this path alone.

Moreover, professional advice can be invaluable. A trichologist or a dermatologist specializing in hair loss can offer tailored advice and treatment plans. They can help identify any underlying issues contributing to hair changes and recommend an effective, personalized strategy to address them.

At the same time, it's an opportunity to redefine what beauty means to you. Many women find that menopause, with all its challenges, brings a chance to experiment with new hairstyles, colours, or even bold cuts that they might not have considered previously. It's a time for reinvention and embracing a new aesthetic that celebrates where you are in life.

Understanding the natural cycle of hair growth and shedding is also key. Hair grows in phases, and during menopause, the growth phase may shorten, leading to thinner, shorter hair. Being patient and gentle with yourself and your hair is paramount during this time of change.

It's also worth considering lifestyle factors that impact hair health. Stress, lack of sleep, and smoking can all contribute to hair thinning. Incorporating stress-reduction techniques, ensuring adequate sleep, and adopting a healthier lifestyle can all have positive impacts on your hair.

Moreover, don't underestimate the power of a good haircut. A style that suits your hair's texture and volume can make a tremendous difference in how full and vibrant your hair appears. A skilled hairstylist can work wonders in creating the illusion of thickness and movement.

Lastly, embracing the grays can be a liberating experience. For many, menopause is a time to celebrate maturity and the beauty of natural changes. Silver strands can be a sign of wisdom, elegance, and a life well-lived. With the right care, gray hair can be just as healthy, shiny, and stunning as coloured hair.

The journey through menopause is uniquely personal, with each woman experiencing a different set of challenges and triumphs. When it comes to hair health, the key is to approach it with kindness, patience, and a willingness to adapt. By taking proactive steps to care for your hair, seeking support when needed, and embracing the beauty of change, you can navigate this phase with confidence and grace.

Remember, menopause is not just an end to fertility but a gateway to a new era of freedom and self-discovery. Your hair, like your journey, is a canvas ripe for experimentation and redefinition. Embrace this time to explore and celebrate the unique beauty of this transformative stage.

Chapter 14:
The Genitourinary Syndrome of Menopause (GSM)

As we continue on our journey of embracing menopause as a transformative experience, it's imperative to address a topic that often remains whispered about, yet impacts many—The Genitourinary Syndrome of Menopause (GSM). This condition, encompassing a range of symptoms related to the genitourinary tract, can significantly affect one's quality of life, comfort, and intimacy. While it might seem daunting or embarrassing to broach, understanding GSM is a crucial step towards reclaiming your bodily autonomy and comfort during menopause.

GSM often flies under the radar, leaving women to suffer in silence as they experience vaginal dryness, discomfort during intercourse, urinary urgency, and recurrent urinary tract infections. These symptoms are not mere inconveniences; they represent a profound change in the genitourinary tissues caused by the decline in estrogen levels that accompany menopause. Yet, with knowledge comes power—the power to manage, mitigate, and even prevent the discomforts of GSM.

Empowering yourself with information is your first line of defense. Understanding the physiological changes that drive GSM can demystify the experience, allowing for a proactive approach to managing symptoms. Treatment options range from over-the-counter lubricants and moisturizers that can alleviate vaginal dryness, to prescription medications and therapies that can rejuvenate the genitourinary tissues. Each woman's journey through GSM is unique, and so should be her treatment plan. It's about enhancing comfort, not just with medication, but also by fostering open, honest conversations with healthcare providers and partners alike.

But managing GSM goes beyond physical interventions. It's also about nurturing self-love and patience. Reconnecting with your body, exploring what feels good, and communicating your needs and boundaries with your partner can transform your experience of intimacy during menopause. Remember, experiencing GSM does not mark the end of your sexual wellbeing but rather invites a new phase of exploration and adaptation.

In essence, navigating through the Genitourinary Syndrome of Menopause is not solely about addressing physical symptoms but is also an exercise in self-compassion, communication, and education. With the right knowledge and resources, you can turn GSM from a taboo subject into a manageable aspect of your menopause transition. The journey through menopause is indeed a holistic one, integrating the physical, emotional, and mental transformations to embrace a stronger, more empowered self.

Understanding GSM

Embarking on the journey through menopause is akin to navigating a rich tapestry of changes, each thread intertwined with the next, creating a picture that is unique to every woman. At the heart of this transformation lies the Genitourinary Syndrome of Menopause (GSM), a term that may not be familiar to many, but is central to understanding the shifts occurring within your body. This section aims to demystify GSM, providing you with the knowledge and understanding to embrace these changes with confidence and grace.

GSM encompasses a range of symptoms and changes affecting the genital, urinary, and sexual health of women passing through menopause. It's a direct result of the decrease in estrogen levels, a hormone that has played a vital role in your body's function throughout your reproductive years. As these levels decline, you may notice a variety of symptoms, including vaginal dryness, irritation, discomfort during intercourse, and urinary symptoms such as urgency or increased frequency. It's a condition that affects up to half of all menopausal women, yet is often shrouded in silence due to embarrassment or a lack of awareness.

The importance of understanding GSM lies not just in the ability to identify symptoms, but in recognizing that these changes are a normal part of the menopause transition. They are not signs of aging to be ashamed of, but markers of a new stage of life to be navigated and managed with self-care and knowledge. By shedding light on GSM, we aim to empower women to take control of their health, seeking advice and treatment options that can greatly improve quality of life during menopause.

One of the key components in managing GSM is opening up conversations around vaginal health. The silence that often surrounds these issues can lead to feelings of isolation or the belief that these changes are something to endure alone. By breaking this silence, we can build a culture of openness and support, where seeking help and sharing experiences becomes the norm rather than the exception.

There are numerous strategies and treatments available to manage the symptoms of GSM, ranging from over-the-counter lubricants and moisturizers to prescription medications and hormonal therapies. Each woman's experience of GSM is unique, and what works for one may not work for another, highlighting the importance of personalized advice and treatment from healthcare professionals.

In addition to medical treatments, lifestyle changes can also play a significant role in managing GSM symptoms. Regular physical activity, a balanced diet rich in phytoestrogens and essential nutrients, and smoking cessation can all contribute to alleviating symptoms.

Moreover, nurturing your mental and emotional health during this time can also impact your physical wellbeing, showcasing the intricate connection between mind and body.

Sexual health and intimacy are also integral aspects of GSM. Changes in libido and sexual discomfort can strain relationships and impact self-esteem. It's crucial to communicate openly with your partner about your needs and concerns, exploring new dimensions of intimacy and connection that accommodate the changes in your body. Remember, intimacy is not just a physical act but an emotional bond that can be expressed in myriad ways.

Understanding GSM also requires a change in perspective, reframing this period not as a loss, but as an opportunity for growth and self-discovery. It's a time to reassess your needs, to nurture your health holistically, and to emerge with a deeper understanding and appreciation of your body's strength and resilience.

Furthermore, acknowledging and addressing GSM can play a pivotal role in empowering women to advocate for their health. Knowledge is power, and equipped with an understanding of GSM, women can confidently navigate the healthcare system, seeking the support and treatments they need and deserve.

While GSM may be a common syndrome, its impact on each woman's life is distinctly personal. Sharing stories and experiences can offer valuable insights and foster a sense of community and solidarity among menopausal women. By listening and learning from one another, we can dismantle the stigma surrounding menopause and GSM, creating a more informed and supportive environment for all women.

In conclusion, understanding GSM is not just about recognising symptoms but about embracing menopause as a natural and transformative phase of life. With the right knowledge, support, and care, you can navigate this journey with confidence, shaping a menopause experience that is positive, empowering, and uniquely yours. Let this understanding of GSM be a stepping-stone to embracing the nuances of menopause, approaching each change and challenge with strength, grace, and resilience.

Remember, you're not alone on this journey. Arm yourself with knowledge, seek support when you need it, and most importantly, be kind to yourself as you navigate the landscape of menopause. Here's to embracing the transformations within, cultivating a life of wellbeing, and stepping into this new chapter with joy and confidence.

Managing Symptoms and Enhancing Comfort

When we embark on the journey of menopause, particularly in navigating the Genitourinary Syndrome of Menopause (GSM), understanding and managing symptoms is paramount to enhancing our comfort and overall quality of life. GSM, while often not talked about as much as hot flushes or night sweats, affects a significant number of women going through menopause. It encompasses a range of symptoms including vaginal dryness, discomfort during intercourse, urinary incontinence, and frequent urinary tract infections, which can significantly impact daily life and intimate relationships.

First and foremost, it's crucial to approach GSM with a mindset of care and attention, rather than one of embarrassment or silence. Acknowledging the changes your body is going through is the first step towards finding relief. Many women find solace in knowing that what they're experiencing is a common part of the menopausal transition and that solutions are available.

Staying hydrated is a simple yet effective strategy for managing vaginal dryness. Water intake can help maintain the body's overall hydration, including that of mucosal surfaces. Additionally, using vaginal moisturisers and lubricants can provide both immediate relief and long-term benefits. These products can help restore vaginal moisture and elasticity, making sexual activity more comfortable and reducing overall discomfort.

Regular pelvic floor exercises, often referred to as Kegel exercises, can be incredibly effective in managing urinary incontinence. By strengthening the pelvic floor muscles, you can gain greater control over bladder function. These exercises are discreet, can be done anytime, anywhere, and the benefits extend well beyond managing GSM symptoms.

For those experiencing more severe symptoms, it's worth discussing with a healthcare provider the options available, such as topical oestrogen therapy. These treatments can significantly alleviate symptoms of GSM by replenishing some of the oestrogen that the body lacks during menopause, directly addressing the root cause of many GSM symptoms.

Diet also plays a pivotal role in managing menopausal symptoms. Consuming a balanced diet rich in omega-3 fatty acids, antioxidants, vitamins, and minerals can aid in maintaining healthy mucous membranes and may contribute to reducing the severity of GSM symptoms. Foods such as flax seeds, salmon, and leafy greens are excellent additions to your diet.

Physical activity is another cornerstone of managing GSM. Regular exercise can improve blood flow, boost mood, and enhance overall physical health, which in turn can mitigate some of the discomforts associated with GSM. Whether it's yoga, brisk walking, or cycling, finding an activity you enjoy can make a significant difference.

It's also beneficial to explore alternative therapies, such as acupuncture or mindfulness meditation. These practices can reduce stress levels, which may have a positive impact on the frequency and severity of GSM symptoms. Stress is known to exacerbate menopausal symptoms, so finding effective ways to manage stress is crucial.

Communication with your partner is key when it comes to managing GSM's impact on your intimate life. Having an open and honest dialogue about what you're experiencing can help foster understanding and patience, and together, you can explore ways to maintain intimacy and connection.

Joining a support group or online community can provide not only practical advice but also emotional support from those undergoing similar experiences. Sharing stories and solutions can be incredibly empowering and reduce the feeling of isolation that some women feel during this transition.

Sleep quality can also affect the severity of GSM symptoms. Since poor sleep can enhance stress and thus exacerbate GSM, striving for good sleep hygiene is essential. This includes establishing a regular sleep schedule, creating a restful environment, and maybe incorporating relaxation techniques into your bedtime routine.

Remember, the goal isn't just to manage symptoms but to enhance your overall comfort and wellbeing. It's about finding what works for you, giving yourself grace, and understanding that it's okay to seek help. Menopause is not just a series of symptoms to endure but a phase of life where you can thrive.

Lastly, staying informed and proactive about your health during menopause is essential. Regular check-ups with your healthcare provider, staying up to date with the latest research and treatments, and advocating for what you need are all crucial steps in managing GSM effectively.

In conclusion, while GSM can be a challenging aspect of menopause, it's crucial to remember that you're not alone, and there are multiple strategies and resources available to help you manage symptoms and enhance your comfort. By taking a holistic approach to your wellbeing, prioritising self-care, and seeking support when needed, you can navigate this stage with grace, strength, and confidence.

Embracing menopause as a natural and empowering stage of life enables us to approach its challenges not as burdens but as opportunities for growth and self-discovery. With the right information, support, and attitude, managing GSM can become just one part of a rewarding journey towards embracing renewal with joy and confidence.

Chapter 15:
Mental Fitness: Keeping the Mind Sharp

The journey through menopause is not just a physical one; it's a mental marathon too, challenging us in ways we might not anticipate. As we turn the pages of this transformative chapter, it's crucial to underline the significance of mental fitness — a beacon guiding us through the fog of forgetfulness and dips in concentration that often accompany menopause. Mental agility is our ally, empowering us to navigate cognitive changes with grace and to keep the brilliant spark of our minds alight. Engaging regularly in mental exercises and activities not only hones our wit but also fortifies our cognitive reserves, offering a robust defense against the natural ebbs and flows of memory and attention during this period. In embracing strategies that range from puzzle-solving to new language learning, we are not merely surviving; we are thriving, turning the tide of menopause into an opportunity for mental expansion and revitalisation. It's a moment to reconnect with the joy of life-long learning, to delight in the challenge of mental gymnastics, and to elevate our cognitive wellbeing to unprecedented heights. Let's embark on this journey with a firm resolve to keep our minds sharp, recognising that mental fitness is not a luxury, but a necessity for a vibrant, fulfilling menopause transition.

Cognitive Changes and How to Address Them

In embarking on this chapter, we're diving deep into a realm that might seem daunting at first glance - the cognitive shifts that come hand in hand with menopause. It's a topic shrouded in misunderstanding, often overlooked in the broader conversation on menopause. Yet, understanding these changes is a pivotal piece of the puzzle in staying mentally fit and embracing this transformative phase of life with open arms.

The truth is, as we navigate through menopause, our brain isn't exempt from the tidal wave of changes happening within our bodies. We might find our sharp wit a hair slower or our once formidable memory taking momentary lapses. These aren't signs of decline but rather natural shifts as our bodies recalibrate to a new hormonal landscape. And here's the liberating part - there's so much we can do to address and even harness these changes.

At the heart of understanding cognitive changes is acknowledging the role of hormones. Oestrogen and progesterone aren't just involved in our reproductive cycle; they have a hand in regulating neurotransmitters that influence mood, memory, and cognitive function. As these hormone levels fluctuate and eventually decrease during menopause, it's not unusual to experience brain fog, forgetfulness, or difficulty concentrating.

But let's pivot from understanding to action - to strategies that not only address cognitive shifts but might also improve mental agility. Engaging regularly in mental exercises is a powerful tool. These don't need to be elaborate; puzzles, learning a new language, or even changing your daily routines can stimulate the brain and foster neural flexibility.

Nutrition also plays a crucial role in our cognitive health. A diet rich in omega-3 fatty acids, antioxidants, and vitamins can support brain function. Incorporating foods like oily fish, berries, nuts, and leafy greens into your diet can be a simple yet impactful step towards supporting your cognitive health.

Physical exercise is another cornerstone of mental fitness. It boosts blood flow to the brain, encourages the growth of new brain cells, and reduces stress hormones. Consistently integrating aerobic exercises like walking, cycling, or swimming into your routine can yield significant cognitive benefits.

Sleep is our brain's time to rest, heal, and consolidate memories from the day. Ensuring you're getting quality sleep is paramount for cognitive health. Strategies for improving sleep include establishing a regular sleep schedule, creating a restful environment, and possibly exploring relaxation techniques before bed to enhance sleep quality.

Mindfulness and stress reduction techniques can also play a significant role. Chronic stress can take a toll on cognitive function, so incorporating practices like meditation, yoga, or deep-breathing exercises can help protect your mental sharpness by lowering stress levels.

Beyond individual strategies, fostering social connections is invaluable. Engaging in meaningful conversations, participating in group activities or simply spending time with loved ones can stimulate the brain and ward off feelings of isolation, which can impact cognitive health.

For those experiencing more pronounced cognitive changes, it's important to consult with a healthcare provider. They can offer guidance tailored to your specific situation, including exploring hormone replacement therapy (HRT), which for some women can help mitigate cognitive symptoms associated with menopause.

This journey through menopause is as much about embracing change as it is about empowerment. Understanding the cognitive shifts that occur is the first step. Taking action through lifestyle changes, mental exercises, and possibly medical treatments not only addresses these shifts but can also lead to a period of profound mental rejuvenation.

Menopause offers an opportunity to reconnect with ourselves, to tune in to what our bodies and minds need. It's a call to nurture our cognitive health with as much care as we do our physical wellbeing. By embracing these strategies, we're not just navigating menopause; we're setting the stage for a mentally vibrant chapter of our lives.

Let's remember, menopause is not an end but a beginning - a chance to reinvent ourselves, armed with knowledge and strategies to flourish. Cognitive changes are but one piece of the menopause puzzle, and with the right approach, we can turn this phase into an era of mental empowerment and clarity.

To all women embarking on or navigating through menopause, know that your cognitive health is in your hands. Armed with understanding and proactive strategies, you can not only address cognitive changes but also enhance your mental acuity. It's a pathway to not just surviving menopause but thriving through it, with your mind sharper and more vibrant than ever.

Mental Exercises and Activities

Maintaining our mental agility becomes ever more important as we navigate through menopause. The myriad changes our bodies and minds go through during this pivotal time can indeed be challenging, but with the right strategies, we can turn them into opportunities for growth and empowerment. This section delves into a variety of mental exercises and activities designed to keep our minds sharp and resilient.

Firstly, it's essential to understand that mental exercises aren't merely about staving off cognitive decline. They're about enhancing our current mental state, boosting creativity, improving problem-solving skills, and fostering a greater sense of well-being. The activities recommended here are tailored specifically with these goals in mind, ensuring that we can approach them with both ease and enthusiasm.

Crossword puzzles and Sudoku are more than just quaint pastimes. Engaging in these kinds of problem-solving activities daily can significantly sharpen our cognitive abilities. They challenge our brains, improve our vocabulary and numerical skills, and there's a satisfying sense of accomplishment with each puzzle solved. But, beyond these more traditional forms of mental exercise, there are plenty of innovative approaches to keep our minds engaged.

Learning a new language, for example, is not just a means of enhancing communication skills; it's a profound exercise in mental agility. It necessitates the memorisation of vocabulary, the understanding of grammatical structures, and the ability to think and translate thoughts on the spot – all of which serve to reinforce neural pathways and improve cognitive function.

In similar fashion, taking up a musical instrument can be tremendously beneficial. Reading music, coordinating hand movements, listening, and creating melodies; all stimulate different areas of the brain, fostering neural diversity. Plus, the emotional connection to music can be a powerful source of stress relief.

Engaging in regular writing activities, whether journaling, creative writing, or even letter writing, can help hone communication skills, offer emotional release, and stimulate creativity. Writing encourages reflection, imagination, and can be a meditative practice, allowing us to explore our thoughts and feelings in a constructive way.

Mindfulness and meditation have gained recognition for their profound benefits on mental well-being. Practicing mindfulness promotes concentration, improves attention, and helps in managing stress. It encourages us to stay present, fostering a heightened awareness of our thoughts and surroundings without judgment.

Physical activities and exercise are also crucial for mental fitness. Activities such as yoga or tai chi not only benefit the body but also focus on breath control, balance, and mental discipline, forming a bridge between physical and mental health.

Brain-boosting diets rich in omega-3 fatty acids, antioxidants, and vitamins have been shown to support cognitive function. Incorporating brain foods such as nuts, berries, fish, and leafy greens into your diet can complement your mental exercise regime.

Joining book clubs or discussion groups provides an opportunity for social engagement and intellectual stimulation. Engaging in debates and discussions challenges us to think critically and articulate our thoughts, fostering social connections and intellectual growth.

Travelling, even if it's local or to relatively nearby destinations, can serve as a potent mental stimulant. It exposes us to new experiences, cultures, and ideas, pushing us out of our comfort zones and stimulating our brains in unique ways.

Engaging in strategic games like chess or bridge, which require foresight, strategy, and critical thinking, can be a great way to bolster cognitive skills. These games not only challenge the mind but also offer a fun and competitive way to engage with others.

Volunteering for causes that are important to us can also mentally enrich us. It places us in situations where we can learn new skills, meet people from diverse backgrounds, and engage in meaningful work that benefits both others and our own mental health.

Taking online courses or attending workshops on subjects of personal or professional interest can keep the mind active and engaged. Continuous learning fuels curiosity, drives personal growth, and keeps the brain in a state of active engagement with new information and skills.

Lastly, gardening, with its blend of physical activity, focus, and connection to nature, provides a therapeutic and calming effect. It requires planning, problem-solving, and fosters a sense of accomplishment and nurturing.

As we journey through menopause, embracing mental fitness activities isn't merely about preserving cognitive function; it's about enriching our lives, fostering connections, and embracing this transformative period with vigour and grace. By incorporating these exercises and activities into our daily lives, we prepare ourselves not only to meet the challenges head-on but also to flourish during this significant life transition.

Chapter 16:
Relationships and Communication

In the realm of transformation that menopause ushers in, the dynamics of our relationships and how we communicate within them can take on new forms and meanings. This stage of life, often misconceived as a phase of decline, is, in fact, a potent time for cultivating deeper connections and articulating our needs and boundaries with clearer, more confident voices. As we transition, it's not uncommon for shifts in our intimate relationships to surface, reflecting the changes happening within us. Embracing these shifts doesn't have to be daunting; rather, it offers a unique opportunity to reforge bonds on terms that acknowledge our evolving selves.

Effective communication, particularly about what we're experiencing, becomes pivotal. It's about expressing ourselves honestly and transparently, a skill that might have been overlooked in earlier life phases due to societal expectations or personal apprehensions. Now is the time to assert what truly matters to us, be it in our personal relationships or wider social interactions. Establishing clear boundaries is equally important, and menopause provides a backdrop against which we can reassess and assert limits that honour our current state of being.

This chapter will guide you through navigating changes in your most intimate relationships, offering insights on how to maintain connection and intimacy even as your body and emotions undergo transformation. Additionally, we will delve into strategies for effective communication. Recognising the power of expressing our needs, desires, and boundaries, we can bolster our relationships and ensure they flourish during this transformative time. Remember, it's not just about navigating the changes; it's about thriving through them, and enhancing our relationships is a crucial element of this journey.

Navigating Changes in Intimate Relationships

As we journey through the transformative stage of menopause, the dynamics of our intimate relationships often experience a shift. This shift can feel disorienting, yet it also offers an opportunity for growth and deeper connection. Understanding and navigating these changes are crucial for sustaining love and intimacy during menopause.

The onset of menopause brings with it a host of physical changes that can affect one's sense of desirability and sexual well-being. The landscape of libido, for instance, might change drastically, leading to feelings of disconnect with one's partner. It's important to acknowledge these feelings and explore them openly rather than allowing them to build unseen barriers.

Communication is the bedrock of navigating these shifts effectively. It's about more than just talking; it's about sharing fears, desires, and vulnerabilities with your partner. This level of honesty can create a foundation for understanding and empathy, transforming challenges into opportunities for strengthening your bond.

Alongside communication, redefining intimacy plays a pivotal role. Physical closeness is just one aspect of intimacy; emotional and intellectual connections are equally significant. Finding joy in shared activities, supporting each other's dreams, and spending quality time together can add dimensions to your relationship that might have been overlooked.

Another aspect worth noting is the fluctuation in emotional well-being during menopause. Mood swings and irritability can strain the most solid relationships. Recognising that these are symptoms of a biological transition—not indicators of the relationship's quality—can help in managing reactions and responses more gracefully.

Sensitivity from a partner is invaluable during this time. Partners who educate themselves about menopause can better support their loved ones. This understanding can foster patience and compassion, reducing the chances of misunderstandings and conflict.

Physical changes such as vaginal dryness and discomfort during sex can be distressing. However, these are not insurmountable. Exploring solutions together, such as lubricants or hormone therapy, and being open to trying new forms of physical affection, can enhance closeness and comfort.

Reviving intimacy often requires a rekindling of romance. Small gestures, appreciation, and dedicating time to be together can reignite feelings of love and attraction. Remember, romance doesn't always need grand gestures; its beauty often lies in the simplicity and thoughtfulness of everyday acts of love.

Couples should also be mindful of the external pressures that can impact their relationship. Societal stereotypes and misconceptions about menopause can lead to unnecessary stress. Rejecting these stereotypes and focusing on your unique relationship dynamic is key to maintaining a strong connection.

Seeking professional support can also be beneficial. Couples therapy or counselling can offer guidance and strategies for adjusting to these changes. A fresh perspective might be what you need to navigate through this period smoothly.

It's essential, too, to nurture relationships with self-compassion. Menopause can sometimes affect self-esteem and body image, impacting how one feels in a relationship. Cultivating a loving relationship with oneself can enhance the capacity to engage positively in intimate relationships.

Exploring new activities together can also be a wonderful way to adapt to changes. Whether it's a new hobby, exercise, or learning something new, shared experiences can bring excitement and novelty to the relationship, enriching it further.

Sexuality during menopause may evolve, but it doesn't diminish. Opening up to new ways of experiencing and expressing sexuality can bring unexpected joy and satisfaction into the relationship. It's about exploring new territories of intimacy together, guided by mutual respect and understanding.

It's also vital to celebrate the milestones and embrace the positives that come with menopause. This period of transition is a testament to the resilience and strength of both partners. Recognising and commemorating this journey can foster a deep appreciation for each other and the life you've built together.

Ultimately, navigating changes in intimate relationships during menopause is about patience, love, and growth. By embracing these changes as opportunities to deepen your connection, you can transform this journey into an enriching experience that brings you and your partner closer than ever before.

Effective Communication: Expressing Needs and Boundaries

In the tapestry of relationships, the thread of communication weaves intricate patterns that can define the strength and beauty of the connection. It's paramount, especially during the transformative stage of menopause, to grasp the art of expressing needs and setting boundaries. This act of disclosure is not merely about speaking but engaging in a profound exchange of understanding and respect.

At the heart of effective communication lies the courage to voice your innermost needs. Menopause is a journey marked by physical and emotional shifts that can feel overwhelming. It's a period when your body redefines itself, and with it, your needs may transform. Articulating these changes to your partner, family, and friends is essential. It's about sharing not just the facts but the feelings accompanying this phase. This open dialogue fosters a deeper bond, creating a shared path through this season of change.

Setting boundaries is equally crucial. It's about asserting your space to navigate this transition on your terms. Boundaries are not walls but bridges—connections that respect your autonomy while inviting others into your experience with empathy and kindness. Whether it's needing time alone, declining social invitations, or setting limits on emotional labour, clarifying these boundaries enhances mutual respect and understanding.

Underpinning these conversations is the act of active listening. This means not just hearing but absorbing the words, emotions, and unspoken feelings of those around you. When we listen deeply, we create a reflective space that acknowledges the other's perspective, fostering a sense of being heard and valued. This mutual exchange elevates the dialogue, making it more inclusive and empathetic.

Effective communication also demands patience. There will be moments of misinterpretation and frustration. Recognising that understanding often requires time and multiple conversations can set a more forgiving landscape for these discussions. Patience with yourself and others allows the conversation to evolve naturally, without the pressure of immediate resolution.

Embracing vulnerability is another cornerstone. Sharing your fears, uncertainties, and the sometimes tumultuous emotions that accompany menopause can feel daunting. Yet, it's this act of openness that invites connection. Vulnerability is a strength, not a weakness. It signals to those around you that it's safe to share their own experiences, creating a reciprocal exchange of trust and support.

Equally, the language we choose is a powerful tool in expressing needs and boundaries. Opting for "I" statements such as "I feel" or "I need" instead of "you" statements helps in taking ownership of your emotions and avoids casting blame. This approach fosters a constructive environment where discussions are centred around needs and solutions rather than criticisms.

Recognising non-verbal cues plays a significant role too. Communication is not solely about the words we say but also about our body language, tone of voice, and facial expressions. Being mindful of these non-verbal signals, both in ourselves and in others, can reveal much about the unspoken aspects of the conversation, enriching the dialogue with a deeper understanding.

Moreover, navigating conflicts with grace and resilience is essential. Disagreements are natural, yet how we handle them can either strengthen or strain relationships. Approaching conflicts with a mindset of resolution and empathy, focusing on finding common ground, can transform challenges into opportunities for growth.

It's also vital to remember the importance of self-compassion. There will be moments when emotions run high, and things don't go as planned. Being kind to yourself, recognising that mistakes are part of the learning process, and allowing yourself the grace to stumble and rise again are crucial parts of this journey.

Creating a supportive environment for these conversations is key. Choosing the right moment, setting, and even preparing the other person for the conversation can make a significant difference in how the message is received. It's about crafting a space that feels safe and conducive to openness for everyone involved.

Furthermore, seeking external support when needed can provide a fresh perspective. Whether it's professional counselling, support groups, or trusted friends, sometimes an outside view can offer insights and strategies for enhancing communication within your relationships.

Embracing the changes that come with menopause also means revisiting and possibly redefining your relationships. As you evolve, so too can your connections with others, grounded in a deeper understanding and more authentic communication.

At its essence, expressing needs and boundaries during menopause is an act of self-care and self-love. It's acknowledging that your journey through this season of life is unique and deserves to be shared and respected. Through effective communication, you can cultivate relationships that not only withstand the waves of change but emerge stronger, rooted in mutual respect and understanding.

Maintaining a sense of humour can be a salve in these discussions. The ability to laugh together, even amidst the challenges, can lighten the mood and remind you both of the joy in your relationship. It's about finding the lightness in the situation, even as you navigate through more profound topics.

In conclusion, effective communication during menopause is about creating a tapestry of understanding, patience, and compassion. It's a journey that calls for courage, openness, and most importantly, a commitment to growing together through this transformative stage of life. By expressing needs and setting boundaries, women can foster deeper connections and navigate menopause with grace, strength, and a sense of shared experience.

Chapter 17:
The Power of Community

As we've journeyed through the intricacies of menopause, from its physical manifestations to the emotional and spiritual transitions, there emerges a triumphant beacon of light: the undeniable power of community. Within the support and solidarity of like-minded individuals, there exists a reservoir of strength and understanding that can significantly lighten the burdens of this passage. Building a robust support network isn't merely about finding shoulders to cry on; it's about creating a collective space where experiences can be shared, wisdom can be exchanged, and laughter can permeate even the toughest of days. There's something profoundly liberating about realizing you're not navigating these waters alone. Engaging in conversations, whether in support groups or informal gatherings, illuminates the path for learning from each other, offering insights that books and professionals might not provide. The shared stories of triumphs and trials act as a mirror, reflecting the multifaceted experiences of menopause, thereby enriching our understanding and approach to our own journey. This chapter is dedicated to exploring the avenues through which we can connect with these vital communities, highlight the importance of giving voice to our stories, and underline the transformative potential that lies within these communal bonds. In harnessing the power of community, we not only find solace and support but also empower ourselves to navigate menopause with a sense of camaraderie, resilience, and grace.

Building Your Support Network

Embarking on the journey through menopause isn't something one should ever have to do in isolation. It's a profound transition that touches every aspect of our lives, from our physical wellbeing to our deepest emotions and how we perceive ourselves in the world. Recognising the importance of a support network during this time can't be overstated. It's about surrounding yourself with people who understand, who can offer a shoulder to lean on, and who can share the wisdom of their own experiences.

The bedrock of an effective support network often starts with family and close friends. It's about initiating conversations, even if they feel a bit uncomfortable at first. Opening up about what you're going through can bridge gaps of misunderstanding and invite shared empathy and support. Don't underestimate the power of being heard and understood by the ones you love.

However, not everyone has a close network of family or friends to turn to, or perhaps you seek the understanding of those who are going through the same phase of life. This is where support groups, both in person and online, come into their own. They offer a space to connect with others on the menopause journey, to share stories, advice, and laughter, and to feel part of a community.

Professional support can also be invaluable. Whether it's a therapist who specialises in menopausal issues or a knowledgeable healthcare provider, these experts can offer guidance tailored to your individual experience. They can navigate you through the physical and emotional aspects, providing a solid base of understanding and options for managing symptoms.

Informing yourself is another critical aspect of building your network. Arm yourself with knowledge about menopause. Reliable resources – books, websites, podcasts – can empower you to make informed decisions about your health and wellbeing. They can also help you articulate your experiences and needs to those in your support circle.

Creating a support network also means being selective about who is part of it. Not everyone will understand or empathise with your journey, and that's okay. Focus on building connections with those who uplift and support you, and don't be afraid to set boundaries with those who don't.

The workplace is another area where building a support network can make a significant difference. Open dialogues with employers and colleagues can foster an understanding environment where adjustments might be made to ease symptoms, such as flexible working hours or temperature control.

Exercise and hobby groups present yet another avenue for support. Engaging in activities you enjoy can not only improve your physical health but can also connect you with like-minded individuals. Whether it's yoga, painting, or hiking, shared interests can be the foundation of supportive friendships.

Technology also offers unique opportunities for building connections. Online forums, social media groups, and virtual meet-ups can be especially helpful for those in remote areas or anyone finding it difficult to attend in-person gatherings.

Remember, the process of building a support network is iterative. It might not happen overnight, and that's perfectly fine. It's about taking small steps to open up, reach out, and connect with others. The strength of community is not just in the number of people, but in the quality of connections and the mutual support it provides.

Moreover, being part of a support network is a two-way street. While receiving support is crucial, offering support to others can also be incredibly rewarding. Sharing your own experiences can help others feel less alone and may provide them with the encouragement they need to navigate their menopause journey with confidence.

In addition to traditional forms of support, alternative gatherings such as retreats or workshops focused on menopause can offer both educational and emotional support. These settings not only provide valuable information but also foster a sense of belonging and community amongst participants.

Finally, don't overlook the importance of empathetic healthcare professionals. A GP or menopause specialist who is not only knowledgeable but also compassionate can make a world of difference. They are an essential part of your support network, offering medical advice, emotional support, and understanding.

Building your support network during menopause is an empowering step towards navigating this transition with grace and strength. It's about finding your tribe – those individuals and resources that uplift, support, and guide you. Remember, you're not alone on this journey. With the right support network in place, you can embrace menopause as a positive and transformative experience, one that opens the door to a new chapter of life filled with growth, wisdom, and wellbeing.

Sharing Stories: Learning from Each Other

In the labyrinth of menopause, the collective wisdom of women who've walked the path before us illuminates the way forward. It's a journey unlike any other, threading through physical changes, emotional revolutions, and a spiritual awakening to a new dawn. By sharing our stories, we not only find camaraderie but also learn from the diverse experiences that shape our understanding of this transformative phase.

The power of community becomes evident when we open up about our menopausal transitions. Each story is a beacon of hope, a lesson learned, or a strategy that worked. It's in these narratives that we find the strength to face our own journeys, armed with the knowledge that we're not treading this path alone. From battling night sweats to seeking solace in spirituality, the stories of women around us can provide both comfort and clarity.

One profound aspect of sharing our experiences is the demystification of menopause. For too long, this natural phase of life has been shrouded in silence, leading many to navigate its challenges without guidance. As women, when we vocalize our journeys, we contribute to a growing body of shared wisdom that can enlighten others. It's through this exchange of stories that we can debunk myths and shed light on the realities of menopause, making the unknown a little more familiar.

Another dimension of storytelling is the emotional resonance it creates. It's not just about the physical aspects of menopause but also the emotional landscape that shifts alongside. From feeling a sense of loss to the rebirth of a new identity, these stories encapsulate the full spectrum of emotions. They enable us to feel seen and understood, providing a sense of belonging to a larger narrative.

The diversity of menopausal experiences also highlights the individuality of our journeys. While there are common symptoms and challenges, how we navigate them varies greatly. This diversity is a testament to the resilience and creativity of women in finding what works best for them. Sharing these individual paths enriches the pool of strategies and solutions available to us all.

Moreover, storytelling fosters a culture of openness that can lead to greater support and advocacy. By talking about menopause openly, we challenge the societal stigma that has silenced women for generations. This shift in dialogue can pave the way for more support in personal, professional, and medical spheres, enabling a more menopause-informed society.

Listening to each other's stories also broadens our perspective, showing us that while our experiences may be unique, our underlying emotions and challenges are often shared. This realization can be incredibly affirming, offering solace and solidarity in moments of solitude.

The act of sharing is also therapeutic in itself, serving as a form of emotional release and acceptance. Articulating our experiences helps us process our emotions, making sense of the changes we're going through. This cathartic aspect of storytelling can be a powerful step towards embracing menopause as a positive and transformative experience.

Community discussions, whether in person or online, have become invaluable resources. They serve as forums for exchange, advice, and support. From dedicated social media groups to community meetings, the avenues for sharing are as varied as the stories they harbour.

Importantly, sharing stories is also about passing down knowledge to future generations. It's a way of ensuring that the daughters, nieces, and granddaughters who follow in our footsteps are better equipped to embrace their menopausal journey. This legacy of wisdom is perhaps one of the most precious gifts we can offer.

In navigating menopause, we discover not just the power of our own resilience, but the strength found in collective experience. The shared stories of triumph, adversity, and discovery are threads that weave a tapestry of communal wisdom. They remind us that our journey is both personal and universal, an individual experience enriched by the shared narrative of womanhood.

Encouraging one another to share and listen is crucial. It breaks down barriers and fosters a supportive environment that recognizes the value of every woman's experience. This culture of sharing and learning is what transforms the menopause from a phase of uncertainty to a chapter of growth and empowerment.

As we continue to navigate our paths, let's remember the importance of sharing our stories and listening to those of others. In doing so, we're not only enriching our own journeys but also contributing to a greater understanding and appreciation of menopause. It's through this collective wisdom that we can truly embrace this transformative stage with grace, strength, and optimism.

To every woman approaching or experiencing menopause, your story holds power. Share it. Listen to the stories of others. Together, let's change the narrative around menopause, creating a future where every woman feels empowered to embrace this new chapter of life with joy and confidence.

In the end, it's through sharing our stories that we learn from each other, finding common ground and diverse strategies to navigate menopause. This chapter is not just about acknowledging the power of community; it's about actively participating in it. By contributing our voices, we make the journey through menopause a shared, empowering experience for all women.

Chapter 18:
Work and Menopause

Navigating the complex world of work during menopause can feel like a daunting task, but it's also an opportunity for empowerment and advocacy. As we tread this uncharted territory, it becomes clear that the workplace isn't just a physical location but a space ripe for transformation. Managing symptoms such as hot flushes and mood swings requires a blend of practical strategies and open communication. It's vital to foster an environment where these conversations aren't just possible but welcomed. Creating a supportive work environment goes beyond individual coping mechanisms; it involves advocating for policy changes that recognise the unique needs of menopausal women. From flexible working hours to accessible wellness resources, the goal is to shift the corporate culture towards one that embraces inclusivity and health. This chapter not only equips you with the tools to manage your symptoms at work but also inspires you to become a beacon of change, encouraging workplaces everywhere to support women through all stages of life. As we redefine what it means to work through menopause, we open the doors to a more understanding, compassionate, and equitable workplace for everyone.

Managing Symptoms in the Workplace

Navigating menopause while juggling a career can feel like walking a tightrope. But fear not, as mastering this balancing act is entirely within your grasp. Understanding how to manage your symptoms in the workplace plays a pivotal role in this journey, empowering you to not only sustain but thrive in your professional life.

First and foremost, knowledge is power. Educate yourself about the multifaceted nature of menopause. Acknowledging that each woman's experience is unique is crucial. Some might grapple with hot flushes during a board meeting, while others may find concentration lapses an uphill battle during their workday. Recognising your own set of challenges is the first step toward addressing them effectively.

Open, honest communication is your ally. Speak to your line manager or HR department about the adjustments you may need. This isn't about admitting weakness; it's about harnessing your strength to advocate for a supportive work environment. Whether it's requesting a fan for your desk to mitigate hot flushes or seeking flexibility in your working hours to improve sleep quality, small changes can make a significant difference.

Adjusting your workspace for comfort is also key. If hot flushes are part of your menopause tableau, positioning your desk near a window for natural ventilation or keeping a portable fan handy can offer relief. Ergonomic chairs and comfortable attire can also enhance your physical comfort, making it easier to stay focused and productive.

Stay hydrated and nourish your body with the right fuel. Sipping on water throughout the day can help you stay hydrated and alleviate symptoms like headaches and overheating. Opting for balanced meals rich in fruits, vegetables, and whole grains can also support your overall well-being and energy levels.

Mastering stress management techniques can be a game-changer. Stress can exacerbate menopause symptoms, so incorporating mindfulness practices, deep breathing exercises, or short walks during breaks can help mitigate stress levels, fostering a more serene mindset amidst the hustle and bustle of your workday.

Don't underestimate the power of a supportive network. Connecting with colleagues who are going through similar experiences can provide a sense of community and mutual support. Sharing tips and coping strategies can boost not just your morale but also that of your peers, fostering a more understanding and empathetic workplace culture.

Consider the benefits of flexible working arrangements. If your symptoms are particularly challenging, discuss the possibility of flexible hours or remote work options with your employer. Such adjustments can offer you the space to manage your symptoms more effectively without compromising your professional responsibilities.

Exercise and movement are invaluable allies. Incorporate short, brisk walks into your workday or engage in gentle stretching exercises. Regular movement can boost your mood, improve your sleep, and help manage weight, all of which are beneficial for mitigating menopause symptoms.

Keep a symptom diary to track how different aspects of your workday affect your menopause symptoms. This can help you identify specific triggers and consider practical solutions or adjustments. Sharing this information with your healthcare provider can also assist in tailoring management strategies to your needs.

Learning to prioritise and delegate tasks can also alleviate work-related stress, potentially reducing the severity of your symptoms. Identifying critical tasks and setting realistic deadlines can help maintain productivity without overtaxing yourself.

Explore the possibility of adjustments to your workload. If certain tasks exacerbate your symptoms, discuss alternative responsibilities with your employer that may be more manageable. This doesn't mean stepping back from challenges, but rather, strategically aligning your tasks with your current needs.

Investigate whether your employer offers wellness programs that include menopause support. Many companies are becoming increasingly aware of the importance of supporting employees through menopause and may offer resources such as counselling or wellness workshops.

Remember, managing menopause symptoms in the workplace is not just about coping; it's about thriving. By making conscious adjustments, advocating for yourself, and harnessing the support available to you, you can navigate this transition with confidence and grace.

In transforming menopause into a phase of empowerment in the workplace, you're not only enhancing your own life but also paving the way for future generations of women to navigate this transition with greater ease and support. Embrace this time as an opportunity for growth and self-discovery, and let your journey inspire those around you.

Advocacy and Creating a Supportive Environment

In the journey through menopause, the workplace can be a domain of unique challenges. Yet, it's also a sphere where the enactment of supportive measures can yield significant benefits, not just for the individual navigating these changes, but for the collective organisation too. This dialogue is about fostering an environment that understands, respects, and adapts to the needs arising during menopause.

First, it's pivotal to acknowledge that menopause is a natural life stage, not an ailment or a weakness. This understanding forms the cornerstone of advocacy within the workplace. Menopause can affect concentration, memory, and physical comfort. Recognising these as potential outcomes of a biological transition, rather than as professional shortcomings, is the first step towards building a supportive atmosphere.

Communication plays a crucial role in bridging the gap between the experiences of menopausal individuals and the wider workplace culture. Open, honest conversations about menopause should be encouraged, not shrouded in silence. This openness not only educates but also normalises menopause as a part of life, making it easier for everyone to be supportive.

Creating a supportive environment also means adapting workplace policies to be more inclusive of menopausal needs. Flexible working hours and the option to work from home can be immensely helpful. So too can providing spaces where individuals can take a moment for themselves if they're experiencing a hot flush or other symptoms. These adjustments, while seemingly small, can make a significant difference.

Moreover, the physical work environment should be considered. Is the office temperature adjustable? Are there facilities to cool down or have a moment of privacy? Simple changes like these can alleviate some of the discomfort associated with menopause symptoms.

Education also plays a pivotal role. Workshops and seminars on menopause can demystify this stage for all employees, fostering a culture of empathy and support. Knowledge dispels myths and misunderstandings, laying the groundwork for an inclusive environment.

Leadership and HR should actively advocate for these changes. They have the capacity to lead by example, demonstrating that menopause is a topic deserving of attention and adaptation. By doing so, they create a climate where employees feel valued and understood.

Peer support groups within the workplace can be incredibly empowering. Sharing experiences and coping strategies can provide both comfort and practical advice. It helps in knowing one isn't alone in their experiences, creating a sense of community and collective resilience.

Access to health support and advice at work can also be a game-changer. Providing services that give menopausal women the advice and support they need reflects an organisation's commitment to employee well-being.

It's also crucial to remember that each person's experience of menopause is unique. Personalised support plans can therefore be incredibly effective. These plans acknowledge individual needs and demonstrate a flexible and compassionate approach to support.

Advocating for change also means challenging any discrimination or stigma associated with menopause. This might necessitate updates to equality and diversity training to include menopause as an important aspect of workplace wellbeing.

The journey through menopause at work shouldn't be one navigated in isolation. It calls for a collective effort, a nurturing of understanding and patience. When an organisation commits to making these shifts, it doesn't just ease the menopause transition for individuals; it elevates the work environment for everyone.

In conclusion, creating a supportive environment for menopause isn't just about health and comfort; it's about respect, inclusion, and recognition of the value that individuals in this life stage bring to the workplace. The steps to advocacy and support are steps towards a more compassionate and productive society as a whole.

Let this be a call to action for organisations and employees alike to champion change. Through education, policy adaptation, and the fostering of open dialogues, we can transform the workplace into a haven of support during menopause. This isn't just a duty but a profound opportunity to enrich our work culture, making it as inclusive and supportive as it can possibly be.

Remember, the transition through menopause is not just a personal journey but a communal opportunity for growth, understanding, and profound respect. Let's embrace this opportunity together, creating workplaces that shine as beacons of support and inclusivity.

Chapter 19:
Creativity and Hobbies

As we navigate through the transformative journey of menopause, it's crucial to find outlets that not only provide respite but also enrich our lives deeply. Creativity and hobbies offer a sanctuary where the turbulence of hormonal changes and life's demands can't reach us. Whether it's painting, gardening, writing, or any other form of creative expression, these activities serve as much more than mere pastimes. They are powerful tools for self-exploration and healing. Delving into creative pursuits allows us to tap into parts of ourselves that have been long neglected or undiscovered. It's about rekindling those flames of passion that life's routines have perhaps dimmed. This chapter aims to guide you on a journey to explore new passions or reacquaint yourself with old ones, highlighting the therapeutic value of such engagement. Creativity isn't about perfection or mastery; it's about expression, exploration, and the joy of discovery. It opens the door to a world where the focus shifts from external validation to self-fulfillment and from consumption to creation. Embracing hobbies and creativity during menopause isn't just an act of self-care; it's a powerful declaration of your ability to generate beauty and meaning, regardless of life's seasons. Let's embark on this creative exploration together, finding solace and strength in the beauty that we can create and the hobbies that bring us joy.

Exploring New Passions

In this vibrant chapter of our lives, as we sail through the ocean of menopause, it's vital to remember the importance of nurturing our creative flames. Exploring new passions isn't just a leisurely pursuit; it's a profound journey towards self-discovery and rejuvenation. Whether you've always had a creative streak or you're keen to uncover hidden talents, now is a spectacular time to dive into new hobbies and interests.

The beauty of creativity and hobbies lies in their boundless diversity. From painting and pottery to gardening and genealogy, there's a vast world of activities waiting to be explored. Each hobby offers not only a chance to learn something new but also a unique way to express oneself and connect with others who share similar interests.

Let's not underestimate the therapeutic value of engaging in creative activities. Painting, for example, can be a meditative process, helping to quiet the mind and ease stress. Similarly, writing offers an outlet for expressing thoughts and emotions, a way to untangle the complexities of our experience during menopause.

It's common during menopause to experience moments of introspection, pondering over the paths we've walked and the dreams we've yet to fulfil. Exploring new passions can be a beacon of light during these times, providing a sense of purpose and achievement. It's not about being perfect at whatever new skill we decide to pick up; it's about the joy and fulfillment that comes from learning and growing.

Moreover, embracing new hobbies encourages us to step out of our comfort zones. This can be incredibly empowering, especially at a time when many aspects of our lives are in flux. Trying new activities helps build resilience, adaptability, and confidence – qualities that are invaluable as we navigate the transitions of menopause.

For those wondering where to begin, consider reconnecting with interests you might have put aside over the years. Perhaps there's an instrument you used to play or a type of dance you enjoyed. Alternatively, joining local clubs or classes can offer both a guided introduction to new hobbies and the chance to meet like-minded individuals.

Technology also opens up a wealth of opportunities for learning. Online tutorials, courses, and workshops make it easier than ever to pick up new skills from the comfort of your home. Whether it's digital photography, creative writing, or even coding, the digital realm offers endless possibilities for exploration.

It's worth noting that exploring new passions isn't just about personal fulfillment; it can also have significant mental health benefits. Engaging in hobbies can reduce feelings of depression and anxiety, improve mood, and enhance overall wellbeing. In the context of menopause, where emotional turbulence can be more pronounced, the value of these activities cannot be overstated.

Furthermore, creative engagements can play a vital role in sharpening our cognitive skills. Learning something new challenges the brain, aids in maintaining memory, and slows down cognitive decline. It's a delightful and effective way to keep our minds as agile as our spirits.

Community involvement is another enriching aspect of exploring new passions. Many hobbies can lead to community projects, charity work, or social groups. This not only expands our social circles but also adds a layer of meaningfulness to our pursuits, knowing we're contributing to something larger than ourselves.

It's also important to remember that exploring new passions is a journey, not a destination. There may be bumps along the way, and not every hobby will resonate with us. The key is in the exploration itself, the thrill of discovery, and the joy of giving things a go.

For some, this chapter of life might offer the chance to travel more, combining the love for adventure with learning about different cultures and their crafts. Travel – whether local, national, or international – can provide unique inspiration and broaden our horizons in unexpected ways.

In embracing new passions, we also embrace a narrative of renewal and possibility. Menopause marks not an end but a beginning – a doorway to new adventures, learning, and self-expression. It's an invitation to rediscover who we are and to paint the canvas of our lives with bold, new colours.

As we journey through this transformative phase, let us keep our hearts open to the myriad of possibilities that lie ahead. Exploring new passions can illuminate our paths with joy, creativity, and profound satisfaction. It's a celebration of life, a testament to our resilience, and a tribute to the unending capacity for growth and renewal that defines us. Let's seize this opportunity with both hands and embark on a journey of discovery that enriches our lives in unimaginable ways.

The Therapeutic Value of Creative Engagement

As we navigate the complex terrain of menopause, finding solace in creative engagement can be both a refuge and a powerful tool for self-exploration and expression. The act of creating, be it through painting, writing, gardening, or any form of artistic endeavour, is not merely a hobby. It's a therapeutic journey that can significantly mitigate the symptoms of menopause, both on an emotional and physical level.

Engaging in creative activities serves as a channel for expressing the myriad emotions that accompany this stage of life. It's common to experience a rollercoaster of feelings during menopause, from frustration to elation, sadness to liberation. Art, in its countless forms, offers a non-verbal language through which we can articulate these complex emotions, processing and understanding them in a way that words often fail to capture.

Moreover, creative pursuits introduce a sense of accomplishment and purpose. Completing a painting, crafting a piece of jewellery, or finishing a piece of writing imbues a sense of achievement that goes beyond the art itself. This sense of accomplishment is particularly valuable during a period when many women may struggle with their self-esteem and sense of purpose, as their roles within the family or workplace evolve.

Beyond the emotional benefits, there's also a cognitive aspect to consider. Creative endeavours challenge the brain, keeping it active and engaged. This mental exercise can be a counteraction to the cognitive changes some women experience during menopause, such as lapses in memory or difficulty concentrating. In engaging our creative faculties, we keep our minds nimble and sharp, fostering a form of mental fitness that can have lasting benefits.

Furthermore, creative activities can foster social connections, either by joining classes, groups, or online communities. These social frameworks not only offer guidance and inspiration but also provide emotional support. Sharing the journey of creation with others breaks the isolation that can sometimes accompany menopause, creating bonds of understanding and mutual encouragement.

It's equally important to acknowledge the physical aspect of creative engagement. Activities like gardening, pottery, or dance incorporate physical movement, gently exercising the body and improving flexibility and strength. Even seemingly static activities like drawing or sewing demand a certain level of dexterity and fine motor skills, contributing to our overall physical well-being.

In exploring new creative outlets, we also embrace a mindset of lifelong learning and curiosity. This attitude is incredibly beneficial during menopause, a time when many women are re-evaluating their lives and contemplating new directions. Learning new skills or diving into new hobbies can be incredibly empowering, signaling to ourselves that growth and change are not only possible but desirable.

Moreover, the act of getting lost in a creative process can be immensely soothing. This flow state, where time seems to stand still, and our worries fade away, is akin to meditation. It offers a respite from anxiety or stress, allowing us to emerge feeling refreshed and mentally clear. This mental 'time out' can improve our emotional resilience and equip us to better handle the challenges of menopause.

Creative engagement also encourages us to look at the world differently. It nurtures an appreciation for beauty, detail, and nuance, enriching our day-to-day experiences. This enhanced perception can foster a deeper connection with our surroundings, prompting us to find joy in the mundane and beauty in the overlooked.

It's worth noting, though, that embarking on a creative journey doesn't necessitate innate talent or previous experience. The therapeutic value lies not in the outcome but in the process. The act of creating is a personal voyage of discovery and expression, irrespective of the end product. It's about allowing ourselves the freedom to explore without judgment, and in doing so, finding a path to self-acceptance and inner peace.

Importantly, creative engagement can be tailored to fit into our lives, however hectic they may be. It doesn't require large blocks of time or expensive materials. Small acts of creativity, incorporated into our daily routines, can have cumulative positive effects on our well-being. This accessibility makes creative engagement a practical and powerful tool in navigating menopause.

In conclusion, the therapeutic value of creative engagement during menopause cannot be overstated. It offers a multifaceted approach to wellness, addressing emotional, cognitive, and physical needs. By embracing creativity, we not only navigate menopause with greater ease but also enrich our lives, discovering new passions and possibilities. Let the journey of creative exploration begin, and may it bring healing, joy, and transformation.

As we continue to explore the myriad avenues of self-care and empowerment throughout this book, remember that creativity is not just an activity, but a mindset. It's about seeing the possibilities, embracing change, and making space for new growth. The canvas of menopause is vast and varied, and through creative engagement, we paint our own unique narratives of this transformative time.

Let us not underestimate the power of creativity to heal, inspire, and renew. As we journey through menopause, let the arts be our faithful companions, guiding us towards a fuller understanding of ourselves and the world around us. In the palette of experiences that menopause brings, may we find our most vibrant colours and our deepest sources of strength.

Chapter 20:
Financial Health and Planning

Navigating menopause also means reevaluating and solidifying our financial health and future planning. As we embrace the changes our bodies undergo, it's equally important to ensure our finances can support our evolving lifestyle and ambitions. It's not just about making it through the here and now; it's about weaving a safety net that can hold us through the years ahead. This chapter is your guide to reassessing financial strategies that align with this transformative period. Whether it's rethinking investment approaches, exploring fresh income avenues, or strengthening savings for unexpected health considerations, we're focusing on creating a robust financial plan that supports both your current and future well-being. It's time to approach your financial health with the same vigour and resilience you've shown in every other aspect of this journey. By planning wisely, you're not just securing your future; you're also empowering yourself to face this new chapter with confidence, knowing you're well-prepared for whatever lies ahead. Let this be a period of growth not only personally but also financially, as you step into a phase of life marked by wisdom and strength.

Financial Strategies for This Transition

The journey through menopause isn't merely a biological transition; it's a profound life chapter that beckons a holistic approach to wellness, including financial health. As we navigate through these turbulent yet transformative times, establishing strong financial strategies becomes as critical as managing our physical and emotional well-being. This section is dedicated to empowering you with practical, actionable financial strategies that align with the essence of this life stage.

Let's start with acknowledging that financial health during menopause can often feel like navigating uncharted waters. Hormonal changes may not only affect our bodies and minds but can also influence our working lives, potentially leading to unpredicted expenses for health care or a reevaluation of work-life balance. This calls for a proactive, rather than reactive, approach to financial planning.

First and foremost, assess where you stand financially. This involves creating a comprehensive overview of your income, expenses, debts, and savings. Understanding your financial landscape is the cornerstone of building a robust strategy that supports you through menopause and beyond. Remember, knowledge is power, and in this case, it's also financial security.

Budgeting, while often seen as a daunting task, is your ally. It allows you to take control of your finances by understanding your spending patterns. Tailor your budget to include potential health care costs related to menopause such as consultations, treatments, or therapies. Also, consider lifestyle changes that may arise, like dietary adjustments or fitness regimes, and allocate funds accordingly.

Savings play a vital role in your financial toolkit. An emergency fund, specifically, can be a lifeline during unpredictable times. If you haven't already got one, start building it now. Aim for an amount that can cover at least three to six months of living expenses. This safety net can help you navigate through any unforeseen financial challenges without added stress.

Investing in your health is paramount. Review your health insurance policy to ensure it adequately covers menopause-related treatments. If you find gaps, explore options to bridge them. While it may require upfront costs, prioritising your health today can prevent more significant expenses down the line.

Debt management is also key. High-interest debt can be a significant drain on your resources, limiting your financial flexibility. Crafting a strategy to pay down debt, starting with the highest interest rates first, can free up more of your money for savings and investments in your well-being.

Let's not forget retirement planning. Menopause is a timely reminder to review your retirement savings and goals. Chances are, your perspective on life and priorities might have evolved. Ensure your retirement plan reflects these changes, factoring in longevity, lifestyle aspirations, and healthcare needs. It's never too late to adjust your course for a more comfortable and secure retirement.

Educate yourself on financial matters. Whether it's understanding investment options, learning about tax-saving strategies, or staying informed about social security benefits, knowledge can significantly impact your financial decisions and confidence.

Consider seeking professional advice. A financial advisor can offer personalised guidance tailored to your unique situation, helping you navigate through the complexities of financial planning during menopause with ease.

On the topic of income, perhaps one of the most empowering moves is diversifying your income streams. In today's gig economy, opportunities abound. From freelance projects to consulting roles, consider what aligns with your skills, interests, and work-life balance desires.

An often-overlooked aspect of financial planning is estate planning. This transition period offers a good opportunity to review or set up your will, power of attorney, and healthcare directives, ensuring your wishes are respected and your loved ones are taken care of.

Lastly, embrace technology. Numerous apps and online tools can simplify budgeting, investing, and tracking your financial goals. Leveraging these resources can enhance your financial strategy, making management smoother and more effective.

In conclusion, weaving these financial strategies into the fabric of your menopause journey can not only bolster your financial resilience but also amplify your overall sense of well-being. Remember, this transition heralds a time of empowerment and renewal. By taking charge of your financial health with the same vigour as your physical and emotional health, you're setting the stage for a future that's not just secure, but also abundantly fulfilling. Embrace this chapter as an opportunity to fortify your financial foundations, ensuring a smoother journey through menopause and a vibrant, thriving life beyond.

The path through menopause is as much about transformation as it is about transition. It's an invitation to reevaluate, reassess, and reinvent — not just in terms of health and wellness, but in every aspect of life, including finances. Armed with these strategies, you are more than capable of navigating this chapter with grace, strength, and wisdom. Here's to flourishing in financial health and beyond!

Planning for the Future

The journey through menopause is not just about managing the present but also about casting an eye towards the future. It's a time that brings about reflection on where we've been and where we're headed. Financial planning during this stage of life is more than prudent; it's essential for securing a future that shines brightly with possibilities.

Understanding that our financial health is as crucial as our physical and mental well-being is the first step towards empowerment. It's about making informed decisions that not only cater to our current needs but also anticipate future aspirations. Crafting a financial plan during menopause can provide a roadmap that navigates us through uncertain terrains with confidence.

One of the core elements of future planning is retirement. Many of us dream of a retirement filled with leisure, travel, and pursuits that we might not have had the time for in our earlier years. However, to transform these dreams into reality, it's essential to start planning early. This involves evaluating our current savings, understanding our retirement needs, and putting a plan into action that bridges the gap between the two.

Investment strategies during this time require a fine balance between risk and security. Seeking advice from financial advisors who understand the unique needs of women approaching or undergoing menopause is invaluable. They can provide tailored advice that considers not only the biological but also the emotional and psychological changes occurring during this time.

Debt management is another critical aspect of financial health. It's about understanding the impact that debt can have on future financial security and taking steps to manage and reduce debt as much as possible. This might involve consolidating debts, negotiating lower interest rates, and creating a structured repayment plan.

Insurance needs often change during menopause. Evaluating life, health, and long-term care insurance to ensure they meet your evolving needs is crucial. It's about protecting yourself and your loved ones from unforeseen financial burdens that can arise from health issues or other unexpected events.

Estate planning, though often overlooked, is a critical component of financial planning. It's about ensuring that your assets are distributed according to your wishes and that your loved ones are taken care of. This involves creating a will, setting up trusts, and making advanced healthcare directives.

Understanding the impact of menopause on work is also essential. For some, this might mean transitioning into less stressful roles, reducing hours, or even contemplating a career change that aligns more closely with personal values and lifestyle preferences. Financial planning during this time should accommodate these potential shifts.

Education is key. Empowering yourself with knowledge about financial planning, investment options, and the resources available to help manage finances during menopause is crucial. There are numerous books, online resources, and workshops designed specifically to address the financial planning needs of women in this stage of life.

But planning for the future isn't solely about ensuring financial security; it's also about embracing the opportunities that this new phase of life presents. It's a time to pursue passions that may have been put on hold and to invest in relationships that bring joy and fulfillment.

Creating a budget that reflects the changing priorities during menopause is vital. This might mean allocating resources towards health and wellness, travel, hobbies, or even new business ventures. It's about making conscious choices that reflect your values and aspirations.

One should not underestimate the power of community when planning for the future. Engaging with networks of like-minded individuals who are at similar life stages can provide not only moral support but also practical advice and resources for financial planning.

Lastly, the journey towards financial stability and independence during menopause is a deeply personal one. It's influenced by individual circumstances, goals, and challenges. However, by taking a proactive approach to financial planning, embracing change, and seeking guidance when needed, it's possible to navigate this transition with confidence and optimism.

As we look towards the future, let us not forget that menopause signifies not an end but a beginning—a chance to redefine ourselves, our relationships, and our dreams. With careful planning, the years ahead can indeed be filled with joy, purpose, and financial security.

In conclusion, planning for the future during menopause is an empowering act. It's a commitment to oneself, a promise to navigate the changing tides with grace and strength. By taking control of our financial health, we not only secure our future but also open the door to endless possibilities that await us in this vibrant chapter of life.

Chapter 21:
The International Perspective on Menopause

In embarking on the exploration of menopause's global landscape, it's enlightening to discover the rich tapestry of cultural attitudes and practices that shape women's experiences during this significant life stage. Across continents and cultures, menopause is perceived and handled in remarkably diverse ways, offering us a panoramic view that widens our understanding and approach towards this natural yet transformative phase. This chapter delves into the myriad perspectives, demystifying how societal beliefs can either empower or stigmatise menopause. By drawing lessons from around the globe, we're encouraged to see menopause not just as a 'condition' to be managed, but as a pivotal opportunity for growth, rejuvenation, and learning.

Gleaning insights from cultures that celebrate menopause as a time of increased status, wisdom, and freedom, we can challenge and shift our own perceptions that are often tainted by the stigma of ageing and loss of fertility. Such global narratives remind us of the importance of dialogue, education, and the sharing of knowledge that transcends borders, empowering women everywhere to navigate menopause with confidence and positivity. Embracing a more holistic and internationally informed perspective enables us to create a more inclusive, understanding, and supportive environment for all women journeying through menopause, ultimately transforming this experience into one of renewal and joy.

Cultural Attitudes and Practices

The journey through menopause is as much about the cultural tapestry that envelops it as it is about the individual thread each woman weaves. Across the globe, cultures shape, define, and reinterpret the menopause experience, infusing it with a diversity that begs understanding and appreciation. In this section, we delve into the myriad ways through which different societies perceive and manage menopause, offering insights that illuminate the path towards embracing this transformative stage.

In Western societies, menopause often bears the stigma of aging, marked by a focus on loss—of fertility, youth, and beauty. This narrative, driven by media portrayals and societal attitudes, can cast a shadow over the menopausal transition, fostering feelings of invisibility or decline among many women. However, there's a burgeoning movement that challenges these perceptions, advocating for a redefinition of menopause as a period of empowerment, renewal, and liberation.

Contrast this with the view from parts of Asia, where menopause is approached with a quieter acceptance. In Japan, for example, the experience is less medicalised and more likely to be considered a natural phase of life, with fewer negative connotations attached to it. The term "konenki", often used to describe menopause in Japan, encompasses both the challenges and the opportunities for growth that this time can bring, highlighting a more holistic view of women's health and well-being.

In many Indigenous cultures, menopause is revered, signalling a transition to a more respected status within the community. For instance, among some Native American tribes, postmenopausal women are seen as wise elders whose insights into life, spirituality, and community are invaluable. Their ability to no longer bear children is intertwined with spiritual beliefs and is seen as freeing them to focus on higher communal duties and spiritual practices.

Similarly, in parts of Africa, the cessation of menstrual cycles often brings relief and a rise in social standing for women. In these societies, the end of fertility doesn't signify a loss but rather a gain in status, with elder women assuming pivotal roles in guiding families and communities with their wisdom and experience.

These diverse cultural landscapes offer a stark contrast to the often singular narrative experienced in Western societies. They remind us that menopause can and should be a time of celebration, a rite of passage that carries with it wisdom, respect, and a deeper connection to the cycles of life.

Yet, even within these positive framings, it's crucial to acknowledge that the experience of menopause can vary dramatically. Access to healthcare, education, and community support can significantly influence how a woman navigates her symptoms and their impact on her daily life. In resource-limited settings, the lack of access to menopausal care and information can exacerbate challenges, highlighting the importance of global efforts to improve women's health services at all stages of life.

Moving eastward, we find that traditional Chinese medicine (TCM) offers a unique perspective on menopause, viewing it as a natural decline in "kidney energy" and an imbalance between the yin and yang forces within the body. Treatment and management practices, therefore, focus on restoring this balance through herbal remedies, acupuncture, and dietary adjustments, emphasizing harmony within the body and mind.

In India, the Ayurvedic tradition similarly offers a holistic approach, focusing on diet, lifestyle, and herbal treatments to manage menopausal symptoms. Ayurveda sees menopause as a transition that encompasses physical, emotional, and spiritual dimensions, urging a balance of the doshas or bodily energies, to ease this passage.

These approaches offer valuable alternatives or complements to Western medical treatments, underlining the importance of considering a woman's cultural background and personal preferences in managing menopause. The global tapestry of menopause experiences teaches us that there is no one-size-fits-all approach to navigating this stage of life; rather, it's a deeply personal journey shaped by a multitude of factors, including cultural beliefs and practices.

For women navigating menopause, understanding and respecting these myriad cultural practices can offer comfort, inspiration, and a broader perspective. It's a reminder that menopause is not merely a biological event but a significant life transition that carries different meanings and is experienced diversely across the world.

This diversity also underscores the need for a more inclusive conversation around menopause, one that moves beyond the medicalisation of this life stage to encompass its social, cultural, and spiritual dimensions. By doing so, we can foster a more supportive and empowering environment for all women undergoing this transition.

Moreover, this international perspective urges us to challenge our preconceptions about menopause, inviting us to reflect on our attitudes and how they are shaped by the culture we live in. It pushes us to consider how we can reshape the narrative around menopause in our own communities to make it more inclusive, empowering, and reflective of the diverse experiences of women around the globe.

In embracing the complexities and beauties of menopause as experienced worldwide, we open our hearts and minds to the rich tapestry of womanhood. This, in turn, can enrich our own journey through menopause, allowing us to see it not as an end but as a vibrant new chapter filled with potential, wisdom, and strength.

Let's carry forward the conversation about menopause with open minds and hearts, drawing from the wellspring of global experiences to navigate this natural transition not just with resilience but with joy and anticipation for what lies ahead. Menopause, after all, is not simply a cessation but a celebration of life, a passage to be navigated with grace, understanding, and a deep sense of connection to the women who have trodden this path before us and those who will follow.

Lessons from Around the Globe

As we tread further into the mosaic of menopause experiences, it's enlightening to turn our gaze towards the global tapestry that illustrates how diverse cultures interpret, respond to, and manage this universal phase of life. The ways in which women across the world navigate menopause are as varied as they are fascinating, offering us a kaleidoscope of perspectives and practices. This global voyage isn't merely an academic exercise; it's a journey towards understanding and empowerment, with each culture offering unique lessons on embracing the transformative potential of menopause.

In Japan, the term "konenki" is used to describe this period in a woman's life, translating roughly to "renewal years". It's a beautifully positive framing that contrasts with Western narratives often cloaked in negativity. Japanese women reportedly experience fewer hot flashes, a difference some researchers attribute to diet, rich in soy products, and a societal attitude that views symptoms as a natural transition rather than a medical condition to be combated. The lesson here? Adjusting our diet and embracing menopause as a natural phase could be keys to a smoother transition.

Heading to India, we discover the concept of "vanaprastha", a phase in Hindu philosophy where one is encouraged to turn their focus inward and engage in spiritual practices. Menopause is considered a liberating phase, freeing women from the cycles of physicality, allowing them to explore a deeper sense of self and spirituality. This perspective teaches us the power of reframing menopause as an opportunity for personal growth and spiritual exploration.

In Scandinavian countries, there's a refreshing openness in discussing menopause, with societal attitudes being more accepting and understanding. This openness fosters a supportive environment where women feel more comfortable seeking help and sharing their experiences. The lesson? Cultivating a culture of openness and support can transform the menopausal experience from one of isolation to one of community and shared understanding.

Turning our attention to Africa, in many tribes, menopause is seen as a sign of wisdom and status. For instance, among the Bantu-speaking peoples of Southern Africa, post-menopausal women often assume leadership roles within their communities. This cultural norm underscores the value of respecting and harnessing the wisdom that comes with age, challenging the youth-centric values prevalent in many western societies.

In Latin America, the diversity of attitudes mirrors the cultural tapestry of the region. Nevertheless, a common thread is the role of the family and community in providing support. Discussions around menopause are often intergenerational, with knowledge and remedies passed down from mother to daughter, fostering a sense of continuity and shared experience. This highlights the importance of community and familial support in navigating menopause.

Moving to the Mediterranean, the diet in this region, rich in fruits, vegetables, whole grains, and olive oil, is often credited with easing menopause symptoms. This diet, coupled with an active lifestyle, points to the crucial role of nutrition and physical activity in managing menopausal changes.

In Indigenous cultures, menopause is often regarded with reverence, seen as a time when a woman becomes a 'wise woman' endowed with new roles and responsibilities. In some North American Indigenous tribes, postmenopausal women are considered the most powerful members of their communities. These cultures teach us the vital lesson of valuing the wisdom and strength that come with age, advocating for a shift in perspective that could greatly benefit Western societies.

Across the Middle East, the experience and perception of menopause can vary widely, often influenced by social, religious, and family dynamics. However, a common theme is the value placed on discretion and privacy. This cultural norm teaches the importance of respecting individual approaches to managing menopause, reminding us that one size does not fit all when it comes to personal health journeys.

In Australia, menopause has begun to emerge as a topic of public conversation, shedding light on issues like workplace accommodations for menopausal symptoms. This movement towards recognition and adaptability offers a lesson in advocacy, illustrating the importance of creating environments that understand and support women going through menopause.

Finally, approaching menopause with a holistic perspective is a lesson shared by many non-Western cultures. This approach encompasses physical, emotional, and spiritual well-being, highlighting the interconnectedness of our health and the world around us. It reminds us to look beyond the physical symptoms and embrace menopause as a comprehensive journey of transformation.

Through this global expedition, it's clear that the way we view and manage menopause is deeply influenced by cultural attitudes and practices. Yet, despite these differences, there are universal threads of wisdom, acceptance, and community support that can inspire us all.

By integrating these global lessons into our own lives, we can cultivate a more positive, holistic, and empowered approach to menopause. It's not just about managing symptoms but celebrating this phase as a time of renewal, growth, and strength. Let's take these lessons to heart, embracing the rich diversity of experiences and perspectives as we navigate our menopausal journey with grace, power, and confidence.

In conclusion, as we traverse the landscape of menopause, let each lesson from around the globe light our path towards acceptance, understanding, and transformation. Menopause is not merely a physical transition but a passage marked by cultural, emotional, and spiritual milestones. By embracing the collective wisdom of women worldwide, we empower ourselves to approach menopause not as an ending but as a beginning—a vibrant new chapter waiting to be written with joy, resilience, and strength.

Chapter 22:
Menopause and the Environment

Embarking on the journey of menopause is not just a profoundly personal experience; it also offers us a unique lens to examine our relationship with the environment around us. As women, our bodies are intricately linked to the rhythms of nature, and this connection becomes more pronounced as we navigate the seas of menopause. The quest for balance within ourselves mirrors the global need for harmony with our planet. It's no secret that environmental factors, such as pollutants and chemicals, can influence our menopausal journey, affecting everything from the severity of symptoms to the onset of this life phase. Conversely, our choices during menopause, from the foods we eat to the products we use, have the power to impact the environment in significant ways.

In this chapter, we turn our focus towards understanding how embracing sustainable practices can enhance personal health and contribute to planetary wellness. It's about knitting together the fabric of our daily lives with threads of mindfulness and eco-consciousness. Whether it's by integrating organic, hormone-friendly foods into our diet, choosing natural fibres for our clothing, or even engaging in gentle, earth-kind exercises, we can make choices that honour both our bodies and the environment. This dual approach not only helps in reducing our ecological footprint but also offers us a pathway to mitigate some of the menopausal symptoms exacerbated by environmental toxins.

We'll explore how, by fostering this symbiotic relationship, we can strengthen our resilience against menopausal challenges while actively participating in the stewardship of our beautiful planet. The aim is to empower you to make informed decisions that reverberate with positive effects on your well-being and the world around you. Menopause, therefore, becomes not just a personal transformation but a catalyst for embracing a lifestyle that prioritizes sustainability and health in equal measure. Let this chapter be your guide to navigating this pivotal phase with an eye towards personal and planetary wellness, crafting a menopausal journey that is as enriching for you as it is for the environment.

Personal Health and Planetary Wellness

As we navigate through the transformative phase of menopause, it's imperative to recognise not only the internal shifts occurring within our bodies but also how our personal health interconnects with the larger tapestry of planetary wellness. This section delves into the symbiotic relationship between our well-being and the environment, offering insights into how fostering a healthier planet can contribute to our personal health, especially during menopause.

Firstly, it's essential to understand that the choices we make daily—from the foods we consume to the products we use—have a profound impact not only on our health but also on the environment. Choosing organic, locally-sourced foods can reduce the chemical load in our bodies, a crucial consideration during menopause when our bodies are already undergoing significant hormonal adjustments. Moreover, supporting sustainable agriculture can lessen our carbon footprint, promoting a healthier planet.

Water consumption is another pivotal factor in personal and planetary health. Staying properly hydrated is vital for managing menopausal symptoms such as hot flushes and supporting overall bodily functions. Simultaneously, using water responsibly and choosing eco-friendly household products protect our waterways from pollution, ensuring clean drinking water for all and safeguarding aquatic ecosystems.

Exercise, while beneficial for our physical and mental health, especially in managing menopausal symptoms, can also be approached from an environmentally conscious perspective. Opting for outdoor activities like walking, cycling, or yoga in nature not only reduces the environmental impact associated with gym-based workouts but also connects us more deeply with the earth, enhancing our well-being through the restorative power of nature.

The use of personal care and household products is another area where our health and environmental stewardship intersect. Many mainstream products contain endocrine-disrupting chemicals that can exacerbate menopausal symptoms and harm the environment. Choosing natural, biodegradable products reduces our exposure to harmful chemicals and minimises our ecological footprint.

Moreover, the aspect of mental health cannot be overstated. The tranquillity and sense of connectedness derived from spending time in nature have been shown to reduce stress and anxiety. For individuals journeying through menopause, engaging in eco-friendly practices such as gardening or volunteering for conservation efforts can offer profound mental health benefits, fostering a sense of purpose and belonging.

Reducing waste and embracing minimalism also play a crucial role in this interrelationship. The clutter and waste we accumulate can add stress to our lives and harm the planet. Adopting a more minimalist approach by reducing consumption, reusing, and recycling can help in simplifying our lives, reducing stress, and conserving natural resources.

Transportation choices further highlight the connection between our lifestyle and planetary health. Opting for public transport, car-sharing, biking, or simply walking more can significantly cut down on greenhouse gas emissions and also improve our physical health by incorporating more activity into our daily routine.

The impact of food waste is another critical consideration. Minimising food waste not only supports the environment by reducing methane emissions from landfills but also encourages a more mindful and appreciative approach to food, which can be particularly beneficial during menopause as our nutritional needs and metabolism undergo changes.

Additionally, engaging with our communities to advocate for environmental policies and sustainability initiatives contributes to broader societal health and ecological preservation, creating a healthier environment wherein we can thrive during menopause and beyond.

The concept of "eco-anxiety," the distress caused by environmental change, is becoming increasingly recognised. Amidst navigating the emotional flux of menopause, fostering a positive environmental impact can empower us, turning anxiety into action and contributing to our emotional resilience.

Furthermore, exploring sustainable fashion and beauty routines cuts down on pollution and waste. Embracing these practices not only aligns with ethical consumption but also correlates with a cleaner, less toxic lifestyle that can benefit menopausal health.

Understanding the environmental impact of medication and healthcare products is also important. Seeking out sustainable health care alternatives where feasible, such as hormone replacement therapy (HRT) with minimal environmental impact, aligns our health practices with ecological consciousness.

Lastly, fostering an appreciation for the natural world can deepen our connection to the environment, underpinning the importance of planetary health in our lives. Integrating nature-based practices into our wellness routines can enhance our well-being and nurture our innate bond with the earth.

In conclusion, the journey through menopause presents a unique opportunity to re-evaluate our lifestyle choices and their impact on personal health and the environment. By adopting more conscious, sustainable practices, we not only support our well-being during this transitional phase but also contribute to the health and wellness of our planet. Embracing this symbiotic relationship between personal health and planetary wellness can be incredibly empowering, transforming our menopausal journey into a pathway towards greater health, harmony, and fulfillment.

Sustainable Practices for Everyday Living

Embarking on this transformative journey that is menopause, it's paramount to not only focus on our evolving bodies and minds but also to consider the impact of our choices on the environment. The path to sustainable living during menopause, while seemingly daunting, is laden with opportunities for personal growth and planetary welfare. It's a chance to harmonize our lifestyle with the rhythms of nature, ensuring our planet remains vibrant and healthy for future generations.

One of the simplest yet most profound steps we can take involves examining our dietary habits. Opting for a plant-based diet not only supports hormonal balance but also reduces our carbon footprint. The agriculture sector is a major contributor to greenhouse gas emissions, and by choosing locally sourced, plant-based foods, we're participating in a crucial shift towards sustainability. This doesn't mean a complete overhaul of one's diet overnight but rather integrating more fruits, vegetables, and whole grains into our meals, making a positive impact on both our health and the environment.

Reducing waste, particularly in the form of single-use plastics, is another key area where our choices during menopause can contribute to environmental preservation. Opting for reusable products, such as water bottles, coffee cups, and shopping bags, can significantly cut down on waste. Moreover, selecting products with minimal or recyclable packaging not only reduces environmental burden but often encourages a healthier lifestyle, steering us away from processed and over-packaged goods.

Water conservation is equally vital. Simple actions like fixing leaks, taking shorter showers, and installing low-flow fixtures can make a substantial difference in overall water usage. As we navigate the physical changes brought about by menopause, developing a more mindful relationship with water use can also foster a deeper connection with the environment, reminding us of the preciousness of natural resources.

Another aspect to consider is energy consumption. Adopting energy-saving habits, such as turning off lights when not in the room, using energy-efficient appliances, and reducing heating and cooling demands through improved home insulation, not only lowers carbon emissions but can also result in significant savings on utility bills. Renewable energy sources, such as solar panels, offer a viable alternative to fossil fuels, further enhancing household sustainability.

Transportation also plays a considerable role in our environmental footprint. Whenever possible, choosing walking, cycling, or public transit over driving can significantly reduce one's carbon footprint. For longer distances, car-sharing or opting for vehicles with lower emissions can make a notable difference. This approach not only benefits the planet but also supports physical health and well-being, aligning perfectly with the needs of women experiencing menopause.

Embracing a minimalist lifestyle can also bring about profound environmental and personal benefits. By decluttering our lives and making more conscious choices about purchases, we not only create a serene and more manageable living space but also reduce the demand for resources and energy associated with the production, transport, and disposal of goods. This mindfulness in consumption encourages a focus on quality over quantity, a principle that resonates deeply with the journey through menopause, where introspection and prioritization become key.

The use of natural and organic products, especially in terms of personal care and household cleaning, can significantly reduce the exposure to harmful chemicals and the release of these substances into our environment. During menopause, as we become more attuned to our bodies' needs, opting for products with fewer additives aligns with a pursuit of health and purity, extending beyond personal well-being to include that of our planet.

Moreover, engaging in community initiatives such as tree planting, beach clean-ups, or local environmental campaigns not only fosters a sense of belonging and purpose but also amplifies the impact we can have on our surroundings. This engagement brings to light the power of collective action and the role it plays in driving significant environmental improvements.

Gardening, particularly with a focus on indigenous plants and biodiversity, offers a unique opportunity to contribute directly to local ecosystems while finding solace and connection to the earth. For women going through menopause, this connection can provide immense psychological and emotional benefits, grounding us and reminding us of the cycles within nature that mirror our own transitions.

On a larger scale, advocating for environmental policies and supporting businesses that prioritize sustainability can amplify our individual actions into broader societal change. By aligning our purchases and investments with our environmental values, we signal to the marketplace the growing demand for sustainable practices and products.

Recycling and composting, though often mentioned, are still cornerstones of sustainable living. By diverting waste from landfills and returning nutrients to the soil, we not only mitigate methane emissions but also contribute to the soil's health, enhancing its ability to sequester carbon. This practice, simple as it may be, is a potent tool in combating climate change.

Furthermore, the phase of menopause invites us to slow down and reflect, making it an ideal time to reassess our lifestyles and the legacy we wish to leave. Sustainability doesn't merely pertain to environmental considerations but also to the sustainability of our health, happiness, and the societal structures we are part of. This holistic view encourages a balanced and thoughtful approach to living that can endure through the later stages of life.

Lastly, educating ourselves and others about the importance of sustainable living creates a ripple effect, spreading awareness and inspiring action across communities. Sharing knowledge and experiences regarding simple, everyday practices can empower others to make changes, forging a collective path towards a more sustainable future.

In conclusion, menopause marks not only a time of personal transformation but also an opportunity to foster environmental stewardship. By adopting sustainable practices into our everyday living, we embrace a lifestyle that honors both our health and that of the planet. This synergy between personal well-being and environmental sustainability paves the way for a fulfilling and meaningful journey through menopause and beyond, embodying a legacy of respect, care, and hope for future generations.

Chapter 23:
Preparing for Post-Menopause

As we pivot to the realm of post-menopause, it's essential to recognise this phase not merely as an end to the menopausal transition, but as a vibrant beginning to a chapter replete with potential for enriched well-being and deepened self-awareness. Post-menopause, undeniably, brings its own set of considerations—where the management of symptoms gives way to a broader focus on long-term health and vitality. It's a time where the physical, emotional, and mental investments made during the menopausal transition can truly come to fruition. By now, the tumult of fluctuating hormones begins to steady, offering a newfound stability that can foster clarity and vigor. Yet, this is also a period to remain attuned to our bodies' needs, championing heart health, bone density, and cognitive sharpness as foundational pillars for thriving post-menopause. Diving into this phase with purpose means nurturing these aspects diligently, underpinning a lifestyle that is as much about preventative care as it is about seizing the joy and wisdom accrued through years of navigating life's ebbs and flows. Embracing post-menopause is about honouring the journey thus far while looking forward with anticipation to the opportunities that lie ahead, crafting a life marked by resilience, health, and fulfillment. As we step into this stage, let's carry forward the lessons of self-care, empowerment, and community, creating a post-menopausal life that is not just survived, but richly lived.

Life After Menopause: What to Expect

As we journey through the vibrant tapestry of womanhood, menopause emerges not as an ending but as a powerful beginning. It's a phase that's often shrouded in mystery, yet it heralds a period of profound liberation and introspection. In the preceding chapters, we've navigated the waters of managing symptoms and embracing change. Now, as we step into the post-menopause terrain, let's unravel what lies ahead with optimism and clarity.

The cessation of menstrual cycles is but a signpost to a broader landscape of transformation. Post-menopause isn't merely a biological status; it's a canvas ripe for reimagining one's life. Freed from the cyclical ebb and flow of hormones, many women find a newfound stability in their emotional well-being. It's as though the hormonal rollercoaster has finally levelled, offering a steadier ride.

Physiologically, while the body adjusts to lower levels of ovarian hormones, this is a period to recalibrate one's health strategy. Emphasis on cardiovascular well-being becomes paramount. Adopting heart-healthy habits, if not already in practice, is non-negotiable. This includes regular aerobic exercise, a diet rich in vegetables, fruits, and whole grains, and monitoring blood pressure and cholesterol levels closely.

Bone health, too, demands attention. The decline in estrogen places post-menopausal women at heightened risk for osteoporosis. Calcium and vitamin D intake, alongside weight-bearing exercises, play crucial roles in preserving bone density. Regular screenings become essential tools in your health arsenal, enabling early detection and intervention.

The myth that menopause marks a decline in a woman's sexual life is exactly that - a myth. Many women report an uptick in sexual satisfaction post-menopause. Freed from concerns about contraception and unshackled from the unpredictability of periods, intimacy can be re-explored and redefined on your own terms.

However, it's essential to acknowledge that the body's natural lubrication may diminish, potentially making sexual activity uncomfortable for some. Yet, this too can be navigated with ease through open communication with your partner and exploring solutions together, ensuring that intimacy continues to be a source of joy and connection.

Mentally, the post-menopausal phase can be incredibly liberating. The wealth of experience and insight amassed over the years becomes a wellspring of confidence and self-assuredness. It's an opportune time to reassess one's goals and aspirations. Perhaps there's a latent passion waiting to be pursued or a new skill to be mastered. The landscape is ripe for exploration.

Yet, let's not disregard the importance of preserving cognitive health. Engaging in mentally stimulating activities, fostering social connections, and prioritising sleep are integral in maintaining mental acuity. Embracing challenges, whether through puzzles, learning new languages, or creative endeavours, keeps the mind sharp and vibrant.

The notion of community takes on a deeper resonance in post-menopause. Building and nurturing relationships with friends, family, and peers provide a supportive network that enhances one's sense of belonging and well-being. It's also a fabulous stage to mentor younger women, sharing wisdom gleaned from personal journeys and fostering a sense of solidarity across generations.

With the landscape of relationships evolving, open and honest communication stands as the bedrock of healthy interpersonal connections. Whether it's with a partner, friends, or family, expressing needs and boundaries with compassion and clarity enriches relationships, making them more fulfilling and resilient.

Nutrition remains a cornerstone of health post-menopause. The body's needs evolve, and so should one's diet. Emphasising foods high in fibre, low in saturated fats, and packed with antioxidants supports overall well-being, helps manage weight, and reduces the risk of chronic diseases.

Physical activity transcends its role as a health requirement; it becomes a celebration of what the body can achieve. Whether it's yoga, swimming, cycling, or weight training, finding joy in movement not only bolsters physical health but elevates mood and enhances cognitive function.

In confronting the challenges that menopause may present, resilience blossoms. This resilience, born from navigating the intricacies of menopause, transforms into a formidable strength, empowering women to approach post-menopause not just with acceptance but with anticipation of the wonders it holds.

Lastly, it's crucial to maintain a partnership with healthcare providers. Regular check-ups, screenings, and open dialogues about health concerns ensure that post-menopausal women are equipped with the knowledge and support needed to thrive.

Embracing post-menopause as a period of growth, exploration, and deepened self-awareness opens a world of possibilities. It's a chapter waiting to be written, defined not by societal expectations but by personal aspirations, health, and happiness. As we move forward, let's do so with the confidence that the best years are not behind us but are unfolding with every step we take into this rich, uncharted territory.

Long-Term Health and Wellbeing

As we continue our journey beyond the labyrinth of menopause, we find ourselves stepping into a realm where our focus shifts towards nurturing our long-term health and wellbeing. This chapter is dedicated to enlightening you on how to fortify your health, ensuring you thrive in your post-menopausal years. Let's embark on this exploration together, with the wisdom we've gathered and the strength we've honed.

First and foremost, understanding that post-menopause isn't an end but a new beginning is crucial. The changes your body has undergone during menopause have now stabilised, offering you a platform to build and maintain robust health. A pivotal aspect of sustaining your vitality is through a balanced diet rich in nutrients, minerals, and vitamins, specifically geared towards supporting bone density, heart health, and metabolic function.

Physical activity remains a cornerstone of good health. However, post-menopause calls for a nuanced approach to exercise. Incorporating a mix of cardiovascular exercise, strength training, and flexibility workouts can help counteract the loss of muscle mass, manage weight, and reduce the risk of chronic diseases such as osteoporosis and heart disease.

Mental health, often overshadowed by physical health, demands equal attention. The transition through menopause can bring about changes in mood and cognitive function. Cultivating a practice of mindfulness, engaging in stimulating mental activities, and fostering social connections can greatly enhance your mental fitness and emotional wellbeing.

Another key area of focus is preventive health care. Regular screenings and check-ups become even more important post-menopause. Staying abreast of tests for breast cancer, cervical cancer, osteoporosis, and heart health can aid in early detection and treatment, significantly altering the disease trajectory.

Post-menopause is also a time when many women experience a renewed sense of libido, free from the concerns of pregnancy. Yet, changes in vaginal health can affect sexual comfort. Understanding and addressing these changes, through lubricants or seeking medical advice for more significant concerns like Genitourinary Syndrome of Menopause (GSM), is important for maintaining a healthy and satisfying sex life.

Let's not forget the skin and hair, our body's protective and aesthetic armour. As estrogen levels decline, changes in skin hydration, elasticity, and hair thickness can become apparent. Nurturing your skin with proper hydration, nutrition, and protection, alongside caring for your hair with appropriate products, can help maintain their health and appearance.

One of the most empowering aspects of crossing into post-menopause is the opportunity to redefine oneself. With potential changes in family dynamics, career, or personal interests, this period offers rich soil for planting seeds of new hobbies, passions, and professional ventures. Embrace this as a time of creative rebirth and exploration.

The concept of longevity isn't just about adding years to life but more importantly, adding life to those years. Adopting a holistic approach that encompasses healthy eating, regular physical activity, mental and emotional care, regular medical check-ups, and embracing change, paves the path for a vibrant, fulfilling post-menopausal life.

Additionally, the support of a like-minded community can be an invaluable asset. Whether it's through local groups, online forums, or engaging in activities that connect you with others on similar journeys, building and nurturing these connections can provide emotional support, motivation, and shared wisdom.

Financial health also plays a critical role in long-term wellbeing. The post-menopausal years can be an opportune time to review financial plans, ensuring they align with your life's new phase. Sound financial planning can provide peace of mind, stability, and the freedom to pursue your passions and interests.

Lastly, it's imperative to remember that health is not just a personal matter but also has a global impact. Embracing sustainable practices in your daily life, from diet to material choices, contributes to personal and planetary wellbeing. This holistic health approach ensures that we not only care for ourselves but also for the world around us.

In closing, transitioning into post-menopause opens up a spectrum of opportunities to enhance your health and life's quality. With the right strategies, mindset, and support, you can navigate this chapter with resilience, grace, and vigour. Let this period be a testament to your strength, adaptability, and zest for life, laying a foundation for years filled with joy, health, and fulfilment.

Remember, the journey through menopause and beyond is as much about rediscovery as it is about continuation. It's a time to prioritise your health, explore new territories, and cherish the wisdom that comes with this stage of life. Embrace it with open arms and a heart full of anticipation for the wonders that lie ahead.

Chapter 24:
Menopause and Legacy

As we transition through menopause, we're afforded a unique opportunity to reflect on our journey thus far and the legacy we wish to carve out for future generations. It's a period that brings with it a wealth of experience, insight, and, for many, a renewed purpose. Crafting a legacy isn't solely about material possessions or accolades; it's about the strength, wisdom, and courage we've garnered through life's ups and downs. This chapter delves into the essence of what it means to leave behind a legacy that encapsulates our deepest values and achievements. Through stories of resilience, we learn that every challenge we've faced has the potential to become a beacon of light for someone else. It's about acknowledging that our experiences during menopause—the adjustments, the emotions, and the triumphs—can be alchemised into lessons of empowerment and strength. Engaging with life's pursuits, we're encouraged to mentor, share our stories, and create spaces that nurture the spirit of sisterhood. By doing so, we not only enrich our own lives but also instil a sense of hope and possibility in others. This chapter aims to inspire you to embrace this transformative period as a prologue to a chapter where your legacy blooms from seeds of self-reflection, growth, and the indelible impact of your actions and choices on the tapestry of human experience.

Reflecting on Life's Journey

Menopause isn't just a biological transition; it's a profound journey into a new phase of life. As we navigate through this passage, it's vital to pause and reflect on the path we've travelled so far. This reflection isn't merely about reminiscing the past; it's a powerful tool to embrace the changes we're experiencing and to craft a meaningful legacy as we move forward.

Life, as we all know, is a tapestry of experiences, a blend of joys, sorrows, triumphs, and challenges. Each chapter has contributed to the person we are today. Reflecting on these experiences allows us to acknowledge our strengths, learn from our challenges, and appreciate our journey's unique beauty. It provides a sense of continuity and resilience as we step into this new chapter called menopause.

Menopause often prompts us to reassess our life's priorities and values. As we experience the physical and emotional shifts, it's natural to question our identity, roles, and the legacy we wish to leave behind. Reflection fosters clarity, helping us to identify what truly matters to us now. It encourages us to let go of past expectations that no longer serve us and to embrace our current realities and aspirations.

Moreover, reflecting on our journey enables us to celebrate our achievements. It's easy to overlook our accomplishments in the hustle and bustle of daily life. Taking the time to acknowledge how far we've come not only boosts our self-esteem but also fuels our motivation to pursue new goals and dreams during menopause and beyond.

Our life's journey also encompasses the relationships we've built and nurtured over the years. Reflecting on these connections can deepen our appreciation for the support network that stands by us. Menopause can sometimes strain relationships, but recognizing the value of these bonds encourages us to communicate openly and nurture them with kindness and empathy.

Reflection also invites us to accept and make peace with our challenges and regrets. Life isn't perfect, and we've all faced moments we wish we could change. Acknowledging these aspects of our journey, forgiving ourselves, and learning from them can bring tremendous healing and growth. This process is essential as we transition through menopause, urging us to let go of burdens that weigh us down and to embrace our present and future with hope and lightness.

As we reflect on our journey, we may discover a newfound sense of courage and adventure. Menopause, with all its challenges, is also a time of liberation and opportunity. It's a chance to redefine ourselves, to explore new interests and passions, and to step out of our comfort zone with confidence. This courageous spirit is a crucial part of the legacy we create, inspiring those around us and future generations.

Our reflections can also spark a desire to give back and make a difference. Many women find that menopause ignites a passion for contributing to their communities, advocating for causes they believe in, or mentoring others. This sense of purpose enriches our lives, leaving a trail of positive impact and wisdom that outlives us.

Embracing a mindset of gratitude is another precious outcome of reflecting on our life's journey. Gratitude shifts our focus from what's lacking to the abundance we've experienced and continue to enjoy. This perspective fosters joy, contentment, and resilience as we navigate the menopausal transition and prepare for the stages of life that lie ahead.

Furthermore, reflecting on our journey prompts us to consider our health and wellbeing holistically. Recognising the connection between our physical, emotional, and spiritual well-being encourages us to adopt a more well-rounded approach to self-care. This holistic perspective is vital as we address the multifaceted challenges of menopause and strive for a balanced and fulfilling life.

Reflection also underscores the importance of authenticity. Menopause is an opportunity to shed societal expectations and pressures, allowing us to live more authentically. Honouring our true selves and living in accordance with our values and beliefs is perhaps one of the most powerful legacies we can establish.

Lastly, reflecting on our journey empowers us to embrace change with grace and optimism. Change is an inherent part of life and menopause is a powerful reminder of this. By looking back on how we've navigated past changes, we can move forward with confidence, knowing that we have the strength and wisdom to face whatever comes our way.

In conclusion, menopause is more than a biological milestone; it's a pivotal moment to reflect on our life's journey, celebrate our achievements, learn from our experiences, and craft a legacy of strength, wisdom, and grace. Let this reflection be a source of inspiration, guiding us to embrace this new chapter with joy, courage, and anticipation for the richness it brings to our lives.

As we continue to reflect on our journey, let's remind ourselves that menopause is not an end but a beginning. It's an invitation to explore new possibilities, to grow, and to flourish in ways we never imagined. Embracing this perspective transforms menopause from a phase to fear into a phase to celebrate. Here's to the journey ahead, full of potential and promise, as we embrace menopause and leave a legacy that resonates with strength and beauty.

Crafting a Legacy of Strength and Wisdom

As we journey through the chapters of our lives, the passage into menopause represents more than just a biological transition; it symbolises an opportunity to fortify our legacy of strength and wisdom. Embracing this stage with grace and empowerment enables us to carve out a path that is both enriching and enduring.

Menopause, often cloaked in misconceptions, actually paves the way for profound personal growth and development. It's a time when the wisdom we've accumulated throughout the years comes to the forefront, allowing us to lead with insight and courage. The knowledge we share and the actions we take during this period have the potential to shape not only our own future but also that of the generations that follow.

Building a legacy during menopause involves identifying the values that are most important to us. This could be resilience, kindness, intellect, or creativity—to name a few. It's about understanding our unique strengths and how we can apply them to impart lasting impacts on our families, communities, and beyond.

In this transformative phase, we are encouraged to reflect on our journey so far. Such reflection isn't about dwelling on the past but rather recognizing the challenges we've overcome and the achievements we've secured. This perspective fosters a sense of gratitude and pride, foundational stones for a legacy built on strength and wisdom.

One of the most significant aspects of crafting such a legacy is the empowerment of others. Whether it's through mentoring, community involvement, or simply sharing our stories, we have the power to inspire and uplift those around us. The lessons we pass on—about resilience, about navigating change, about embracing one's true self— these are the threads that weave a lasting tapestry of influence.

Moreover, menopause is a period that prompts us to redefine our priorities. What matters most may shift, and this re-evaluation is essential in directing our energies towards what genuinely enriches our lives and the lives of others. It's about making intentional choices that resonate with our core values and aspirations.

A crucial component of this legacy-building is self-care. Prioritizing our physical, emotional, and mental health ensures we have the strength to pursue our goals and support others. This might mean adopting a balanced diet, committing to regular exercise, finding solace in meditation, or seeking joy in hobbies. A well-nourished self is more capable of nourishing others.

This stage also invites us to cultivate resilience. Menopause can present its set of challenges, from physical symptoms to emotional upheavals. However, facing these with determination and a positive outlook reinforces our capacity to adapt and thrive. This resilience becomes a key part of the legacy we offer, demonstrating that challenges are not just obstacles but catalysts for growth.

Similarly, wisdom in this context isn't merely about the accumulation of knowledge. It's about applying our insights for the greater good, making decisions that reflect a deep understanding of life's complexities. This wisdom enables us to act as beacons of guidance and support for others navigating their pathways.

Additionally, crafting a legacy involves embracing change with open arms. Menopause signifies one of life's significant transitions, and our attitude towards this change can set a powerful example. By meeting this new chapter with enthusiasm and openness, we demonstrate the beauty of transformation at any stage of life.

In sharing our stories, we shouldn't shy away from authenticity. The challenges, the successes, the moments of doubt, and the triumphs—all these elements make our journey relatable and inspiring. Authenticity strengthens our legacy, showing that it's in the mosaic of human experiences that true wisdom lies.

Volunteering and community engagement also offer channels through which we can extend our influence. Active participation in causes we're passionate about not only enriches our lives but also leaves indelible marks on the fabric of society. These acts of service are integral to a legacy grounded in strength and wisdom.

As we navigate menopause, it's crucial to foster connections—both nurturing established relationships and forging new ones. These connections provide us with a sense of belonging and support, vital components of any endeavor to build a meaningful legacy. Moreover, they enable us to exchange knowledge and experiences, further multiplying the impact of our wisdom.

Lastly, envisioning the future we aim to create through our legacy is essential. Setting goals and visualizing the influence we wish to have guides our actions and decisions towards making that vision a reality. It's a process of translating our strength and wisdom into tangible outcomes that can benefit others long after we've moved onto the next chapter of our lives.

In conclusion, navigating the menopausal transition with intention and purpose sets the stage for crafting a legacy of enduring strength and wisdom. It's a journey that asks us to look inward, to evaluate, and to act in ways that resonate with our deepest values. By doing so, we not only enrich our own lives but also inspire and empower those around us, sowing the seeds for a future built on the pillars of resilience, kindness, and insightful understanding.

Chapter 25:
Embracing Renewal with Joy and Confidence

We've traversed the multifaceted landscape of menopause together, exploring its contours from the biological, emotional, psychological, and even spiritual dimensions. With each step, the journey has unfolded revealing both challenges and profound opportunities for growth, transformation, and renewal. Now, as we stand on the precipice of closing this chapter, it's essential to look forward with joy and confidence, equipped with the knowledge and strategies we've shared.

Menopause is undoubtedly a significant life transition, characterised by an array of physical and emotional changes. However, with the perspectives and tools you've gained, this transition can be viewed not as an ending but as a remarkable opportunity for rebirth. It's a time to reconnect with your deepest desires, reassess your health, and reinvigorate your mindset towards living a life aligned with your core values and aspirations.

It's also pivotal to acknowledge the power of embracing change with a positive outlook. The attitude with which you approach this stage can significantly impact your experience. Viewing menopause as a natural, empowering phase of life can transform challenges into stepping stones for personal growth and fulfillment.

Exercise and nutrition have emerged as central pillars supporting your journey through menopause. Tailoring your diet to meet the unique needs of your changing body, coupled with adopting an exercise regime that resonates with your lifestyle, can significantly ease symptoms and enhance your vitality. Remember, consistency is key, and patience is a virtue when adapting to new habits.

Alternative therapies and supplements have also shown promise, offering natural remedies to manage symptoms. As you continue to explore these options, let your body's response guide you. What works for one person may not for another, highlighting the importance of a personalised approach to menopause management.

Medical treatments, including hormone replacement therapy (HRT), offer another avenue for symptom relief, underscoring the necessity of open, informed discussions with healthcare providers. Your journey is unique, and so too should be your treatment plan, designed to meet your specific needs and health goals.

The significance of mental and emotional well-being cannot be overstated. Nurturing your mind and spirit through this transition is crucial. Strategies that foster resilience, such as mindfulness, stress-reduction techniques, and cultivating a strong support network, are invaluable resources. They empower you to navigate this chapter with a balanced and hopeful perspective.

Moreover, menopause presents an opportune moment to reflect on relationships, work, and the pursuit of passions or hobbies that bring joy and satisfaction. It's a time to communicate needs, set boundaries, and deepen connections with loved ones. Emphasising effective communication can lead to strengthened relationships, enriched by mutual understanding and support.

Community plays a pivotal role, offering a sense of belonging and shared experience. Building or joining a network of women who are navigating similar transitions can provide comfort, insights, and encouragement. Sharing stories and lessons learned fosters a collective wisdom that enriches the menopause journey for all.

Looking forward, menopause is also a time to ponder legacy and the imprint you wish to leave on the world. Reflecting on life's journey hitherto, crafting a vision for the future, and taking deliberate steps towards realising that vision can be profoundly rewarding.

Environmental considerations also come into sharper focus, inspiring a mindful examination of how personal health practices can align with the sustainability of our planet. Embracing eco-friendly lifestyle choices reflects a commitment to nurturing oneself and the environment in tandem.

As we prepare for post-menopause, it's critical to anticipate the continuation of life's journey with an eye towards long-term health and well-being. The strategies embraced during menopause can lay the groundwork for a vibrant, healthy future, rich with possibilities.

So, as we conclude, remember that menopause is not just an end to fertility but a dawn of new beginnings. It's a time ripe with potential for redefining identity, renewing commitments to health and happiness, and realising dreams that may have been deferred. Embrace this transition with joy and confidence, knowing you're equipped to navigate the journey with grace, strength, and an open heart.

Finally, let us recall that within every woman lies an incredible reservoir of resilience and wisdom. Menopause is an opportunity to tap into this wellspring, to cultivate a life that resonates with authenticity and vibrance. Moving forward, let these insights and strategies be your guide, illuminating the path towards a future filled with health, happiness, and fulfilment. Embrace this chapter of renewal with open arms, and step into the next phase of your life with joy and unshakeable confidence.

Appendix A:
Resources and Support

At the end of this transformative journey, it's not just about having navigated through the tempest of change but also about the invaluable resources and support systems that have been our lighthouses. In this appendix, we aim to provide a comprehensive collection of these vital beacons. Whether you're seeking deeper knowledge, a sense of community, or practical advice to illuminate this path, you'll find an array of resources tailored to your needs.

Recommended Reading

Knowledge is power, especially when it comes to understanding and managing your menopause experience. With a plethora of information available, it can be overwhelming to sift through what's beneficial. We've compiled a list of seminal works that offer not just scientific insights but also personal stories and practical advice:

- *The Complete Guide to Menopause: Insights and Advice for a Smooth Transition* - This comprehensive book covers all aspects of menopause, from biological changes to emotional and physical strategies for managing symptoms.

- *Menopause and Mindfulness: Embracing Change with Grace* - Combining personal anecdotes with meditation techniques, this book offers a unique approach to finding balance and peace through menopause.

- *Nutrition for the Menopausal Years: Eating Right for a Balanced Life* - A deep dive into how nutritional needs change during menopause and how to adapt your diet to support your health.

These titles are just the tip of the iceberg, but they're a solid foundation for anyone looking to understand menopause better and navigate it with confidence.

Support Groups and Organisations

Finding a community that resonates with your experiences can be incredibly validating and empowering. Here are some organisations and support groups that provide a safe space to share, learn, and connect with others who are on a similar journey:

- **The Menopause Charity** - Offering extensive resources, advice, and support, this charity seeks to empower women through education and advocate for better menopausal care.

- **Women's Health Concern** - A patient arm of the British Menopause Society, this organisation provides confidential advice and support on all aspects of women's health, including menopause.

- **Menopause Support Network** - A vibrant online community that provides a platform for sharing experiences, strategies, and support. They host regular webinars and discussions on various menopause-related topics.

Connecting with others who understand exactly what you're going through can make all the difference. These groups not only offer support but also foster a sense of belonging and empowerment among their members.

Final Thoughts

Embarking on the menopause journey can feel daunting, but you're not alone. Armed with knowledge and surrounded by a supportive community, this transition can be navigated with grace and strength. Remember, menopause is not just an end but a beginning - a gateway to a new chapter filled with opportunities for growth, health, and fulfilment. Embrace it with an open heart and mind, and let these resources guide you towards a future brimming with potential.

We hope this appendix serves as a valuable tool in your journey, providing you with the support and resources needed to thrive during menopause and beyond. Your path may be unique, but together, we can all move forward with courage and confidence.

Recommended Reading

Embarking on the menopause journey can often feel like navigating through uncharted waters. However, the beacon of knowledge shines brightly through the fog, guiding us towards understanding and empowerment. The literature on menopause is vast and diverse, offering insights from medical, psychological, and personal perspectives. In this section, we've curated a comprehensive reading list that serves as your compass through this journey, enabling you to embrace menopause with confidence and grace.

First and foremost, understanding the biology of menopause is crucial. We recommend starting with books that delve into the hormonal changes your body undergoes during this period. These texts illuminate the physical transformations in an accessible manner, equipping you with the knowledge to collaborate effectively with healthcare professionals.

Debunking myths about menopause is another critical area. Reading material that challenges common misconceptions can be liberating. It allows you to separate fact from fiction, freeing you from unnecessary fears and setting the stage for a more positive experience.

The emotional and psychological dimensions of menopause deserve attention as well. Books that explore the impact of hormonal fluctuations on your mental well-being, mood, and self-perception are invaluable. They offer strategies for maintaining emotional balance and embracing the changes in your self-identity with kindness and compassion.

Menopause also invites a spiritual journey, a quest for meaning amidst the transformation. Select readings can guide you in nurturing inner peace and finding deeper significance in this life stage. They encourage reflection and foster a sense of connectedness to oneself and the universe.

Nutrition and physical activity are pillars of navigating menopause with vitality. The recommended readings in these areas unveil the power of dietary choices and exercise in managing menopausal symptoms, highlighting practical advice for integrating these habits into your daily life.

Exploring alternative therapies and supplements can also be beneficial. Opt for books that discuss herbal remedies and supplements with a critical eye, focusing on scientific evidence to help you make informed decisions.

Medical treatments, including hormone replacement therapy (HRT), are complex topics. Choose books that present the pros and cons objectively, providing comprehensive insights into the various options available. This knowledge empowers you to engage in informed discussions with your healthcare provider about the best course of action tailored to your unique needs.

Considering the changes in cardiovascular health and bone integrity during menopause, it's essential to educate yourself on these aspects. Selected readings offer preventative strategies and management techniques, fostering a proactive approach to maintaining your heart and bone health.

The transformation of skin and hair, as well as the genitourinary syndrome of menopause (GSM), are addressed in publications that combine medical advice with practical self-care tips. These resources offer comfort and reassure you that you're not alone in these experiences.

Mental fitness is another key aspect. Engage with books that provide mental exercises and activities designed to keep your mind sharp. They empower you to combat cognitive changes and stimulate mental agility.

The impact of menopause on relationships and communication can be profound. Reading material in this domain reveals insights into navigating changes in intimate relationships and effective ways of expressing needs and boundaries.

The concept of community and the importance of building a support network are explored in readings that emphasize shared experiences. They illustrate the strength found in connection and the enriching benefits of learning from one another.

Lastly, embracing creativity and hobbies emerges as a significant theme. Resources highlighting the therapeutic value of creative engagement during menopause inspire you to explore new passions and discover renewal in self-expression.

In conclusion, the journey through menopause is as unique as you are. The recommended readings in this section provide a multifaceted view, encompassing the physical, emotional, psychological, and spiritual aspects. They serve not just as guides but as companions, offering solace, inspiration, and empowerment. As you navigate this transformative phase, let knowledge be your ally, and remember that menopause is not merely an end but a vibrant beginning.

Support Groups and Organisations

As we journey through the landscape of menopause, it's important to remember you're not alone. Across the globe, countless women are navigating this transformative period, each with their unique experiences and insights. The power of community cannot be underestimated, especially during times of change. In this section, we'll explore various support groups and organisations dedicated to providing assistance, education, and a sense of camaraderie during menopause.

Menopause societies and organisations offer a wealth of information, spanning from medical advice to lifestyle tips that cater specifically to the needs of menopausal women. These institutions often spearhead research, ensuring that members have access to the latest findings and treatments. Joining a society can significantly demystify the menopause process, equipping you with knowledge to make informed decisions about your health.

Support groups, on the other hand, provide a more intimate setting for sharing and learning. These groups, which can be found both online and in local communities, offer a platform for women to voice their concerns, share their stories, and find solace in shared experiences. The empathetic understanding that comes from someone who's walking a similar path is invaluable. It's in these spaces that friendships are forged, providing strength and comfort when it's needed most.

Focused workshops and seminars are other avenues through which menopausal women can enhance their journey. These sessions, often hosted by experts in the field, cover a range of topics from hormonal changes to lifestyle adjustments. They not only educate but also empower participants to take control of their menopause experience.

Online forums and social media groups have emerged as invaluable resources for menopausal women. These digital platforms provide the flexibility to seek support and exchange information from the comfort of one's home. The anonymity of online groups can also make it easier to discuss topics that many find sensitive or embarrassing.

Healthcare organisations and clinics frequently offer support services for menopausal women, including counselling and therapy sessions. These services aim to address both the physical and emotional aspects of menopause, offering holistic support. Access to professional health advice ensures that women are not only heard but also guided through their options for managing symptoms.

Charities dedicated to women's health play a pivotal role in raising awareness and advocacy for menopausal support. They work tirelessly to ensure that menopause is recognised as a significant phase in a woman's life, deserving of attention and care. Through fundraising and campaigns, these charities strive to improve services and support for menopausal women, making a tangible difference in their quality of life.

Educational resources, including books, websites, and newsletters, offer a treasure trove of information. They can guide you through nutritional advice, exercise tips, and holistic practices designed to ease menopause symptoms. Being well-informed boosts confidence and equips you with strategies to navigate menopause more smoothly.

Peer mentoring programs connect those newly navigating menopause with women who have already transitioned through it. These mentorships offer personalised support and insights, providing a guiding light through the menopausal journey. Such connections can be incredibly reassuring, offering proof that there's life – vibrant and fulfilling – beyond menopause.

Interactive workshops and retreats offer unique opportunities for immersion into practices beneficial for menopause management, such as yoga and mindfulness. These gatherings not only provide valuable techniques for symptom management but also offer a collective experience of rejuvenation and bonding with others on a similar path.

Community centres and clubs may not exclusively cater to menopausal women but can offer activities and gatherings that support overall well-being. Engaging in regular social activities can significantly boost morale and provide a sense of normalcy during the transitions of menopause.

Lastly, it's worth considering speaking engagements and conferences focused on women's health and menopause. These events bring together experts, advocates, and those experiencing menopause, fostering a rich exchange of knowledge and experiences. They serve as a powerful reminder of the collective strength and wisdom that can be harnessed to navigate menopause with grace.

In summary, the range of support groups and organisations available to women going through menopause is vast and varied. From providing medical information and emotional support to advocating for greater understanding and better healthcare, these resources play a crucial role in supporting women through this significant life stage. Whether you're looking for advice, companionship, or professional services, there's a community out there ready to welcome you with open arms.

The journey through menopause is deeply personal, yet universally shared. The strength, insight, and camaraderie offered by support groups and organisations can transform this journey into a more positive and empowered experience. By seeking out these resources, you're taking an important step towards not just managing menopause but thriving through it.

Embrace the support available; let it lift and guide you through the waves of menopause. Together, we can turn this chapter of life into one of renewal, growth, and profound transformation.